Congenital Heart Disease
in Adults

Congenital Heart Disease in Adults
A Practical Guide

Andrew Redington
Darryl Shore
Paul Oldershaw

Royal Brompton Hospital

WB Saunders Company Ltd
London   Philadelphia   Toronto   Sydney   Tokyo

W.B. Saunders Company Ltd   24–28 Oval Road
London NW1 7DX

The Curtis Center
Independence Square West
Philadelphia, PA 19106–3399, USA

Harcourt Brace & Company
55 Horner Avenue
Toronto, Ontario, M8Z 4X6, Canada

Harcourt Brace & Company, Australia
30–52 Smidmore Street
Marrickville
NSW 2204, Australia

Harcourt Brace & Company, Japan
Ichibancho Central Building
22–1 Ichibancho
Chiyoda-ku, Tokyo 102, Japan

A catalogue record for this book is available from the British Library

ISBN 0–7020–1913–5

Typeset by J&L Composition Ltd, Filey, North Yorkshire
Printed and bound in Great Britain by The University Press, Cambridge

Contents

Section 4 Specific problems   191

Preface

It would be difficult to write a book on congenital heart disease in adults without reproducing an enormous amount of information already splendidly presented in major textbooks of paediatric congenital heart disease, echocardiography, angiocardiography, transoesophageal echo, etc. This book is not in any way intended to provide an all embracing review of all the issues in adult congenital heart disease. Rather, it is presented as a guidebook. Our aim was to produce a readable text, which allows those who are not specialists in the field, to understand the language and practice of congenital heart disease and how it is applied to those outgrowing their paediatric cardiologist and paediatrician, as they become adults.

There are specialist units concerned with the treatment of adults with congenital heart disease, but they are few and far between. More and more children are surviving early surgery and adult physicians and cardiologists will be encountering these patients more frequently. Not everybody has the time or the inclination to undertake formal training in congenital heart disease, and this book is for them. In a sense, it is a guide as to 'when to refer'. In general, if your patient falls outside the broad guidelines given in this book he or she probably requires a specialist's opinion. A recurring theme throughout the book is that these patients cannot be considered either as larger versions of children with congenital heart disease, or necessarily managed in the same way as an older adult with acquired heart disease. The issues may be quite different, and require specific individualized investigation and treatment. A recognition of one's own limitations is important in any branch of medicine, but is no better illustrated than in the care of adults with congenital heart disease.

ANR
DS
PJO.

Section 1

Functional Assessment of the Adult and Adolescent

1 Clinical Assessment

In collaboration with Dr RH Stables

Introduction

Careful clinical evaluation is central to the assessment of patients with congenital heart disease. Although modern imaging techniques have revolutionized investigation and pre mortem diagnosis, the traditional skills of history taking and clinical examination are far from obsolete.

A congenital abnormality is initially suggested by the clinical history or an abnormal finding on physical examination. A reliable diagnosis can sometimes be made from this information alone, though in modern practice confirmation and detailed characterization is normally sought with additional diagnostic techniques.

This chapter will review the principles of physical examination in adult congenital heart disease. Details of physical signs that are associated with particular diagnostic groups or conditions are included in the relevant chapters.

Organization

Congenital heart disease is a specialist area and many adult cardiologists, particularly those in training grades, will have little practical experience in its assessment. Familiarity with an often complex and extensive past medical history and a clear understanding of the medium- and long-term management strategy are essential for proper case review. Patients may be young and somewhat vulnerable with physical, psychological and social problems. Accurate clinical assessment will necessitate an appreciation of how these and other issues may affect presentation. There is merit therefore in arranging follow-up appointments so that patients are reviewed by a particular individual or one of a small group of dedicated physicians working as part of an established multidisciplinary healthcare team. Clinical teaching should be encouraged within this setting to improve clinical skills and extend experience.

Consultations should be conducted in an appropriate environment. The waiting area may be occupied by patients from a range of age groups and levels of maturity. It is desirable to provide separate facilities for younger patients. Adolescents are often a difficult group to deal with, especially those who have had to cope with chronic illness, disability and sometimes extensive periods in medical care. Such patients often seek a degree of independence and autonomy from their patients and this may require a separate room for physical examination. Chaperons should always be available to assist during physical examinations. Good lighting and low background noise levels are important in any examination but vital in this case. Parents should be allowed in the consultation room but the adolescent patient should always be asked what *they* want.

It may be useful to produce unit protocols that specify aspects of the clinical history and physical examination to be elucidated and recorded at each follow-up visit. These should also provide a schedule for the performance of routine investigations such as blood tests, radiographs, exercise tolerance tests and echocardiography. Audit studies from a number of clinical disciplines have established that the implementation of protocols in this setting has improved standards of care. A protocol is usually required for each diagnostic group but an unusual or complex patient may necessitate an individual schedule.

Detailed and clear clinical records should be kept and the results of key investigations entered in the notes. Changes in diagnosis, treatment or the overall management strategy must be documented. It is important to include details of information and advice given to the patient or to friends and relatives. If possible this should encompass an assessment of their understanding of the situation. Specific areas of concern or unresolved issues should be identified. This will allow future consultations to be conducted on an appropriate level. The findings at, and outcome of, each consultation should be distributed to all professionals involved in shared care.

Initial assessment

A full clinical history should be elicited. Cardiologists normally involved in the care of adults may find it useful to revise those aspects of the history peculiar to the assessment of the younger patient, for example birth details, developmental milestones and immunization history. It is important to attempt to assess the impact of the patient's condition on aspects of daily life. This should include measures of exercise tolerance and work capacity, educational development, social and (if applicable) sexual issues. Important life events should be noted and appropriate advice given, for example, in relation to contraception, pregnancy and genetic counselling (see Chapter 22).

General examination of younger patients should include charting of height and weight against standard reference charts. In the adolescent the development of secondary sexual characteristics should be noted. Adequate exposure (with attention to the protection of modesty) is essential. It is, for example, important to examine the lower limbs and feet with the precision that is often afforded only to the hands and arms in patients with acquired heart disease.

In certain circumstances the bedside clinical assessment can be significantly enhanced with the performance of simple non-invasive tests. An example of this is the assessment of arterial oxygen saturation. Central cyanosis is an indication of arterial desaturation and may be noted when more than 5 g/dl of reduced haemoglobin is circulating. The physical sign is therefore dependent, in part, on the total haemoglobin concentration and may be absent in patients with significant desaturation but reduced red cell mass. Pulse oxymetry now allows rapid, non-invasive assessment of arterial oxygen saturation and can be used both at rest and during exercise. This allows a quantitative assessment of saturation under different physical conditions. Similarly exercise capacity can be better assessed with a variety of tests including a maximal treadmill exercise testing, or a timed walk test. Application of this approach allows a more rational and scientific assessment of disease progression and treatment effect.

Examination of the cardiovascular system

The essentials of clinical examination are common to congenital and acquired disease. Some aspects important in the assessment of congenital cases are highlighted below.

Arterial pulses

The character and force of the pulses must be compared both between left and right arms and between legs and arms. Previous arteriotomy sites should be avoided as the procedure may have caused local arterial stenosis. If the leg pulses are decreased or absent then coarctation of the aorta must be suspected. The origin of the left subclavian artery may be involved to a greater or lesser extent and if this is the case the left arm pulses will also be reduced. Radial–femoral delay is a common finding and, in the older patient, the presence of arterial collaterals particularly in the periscapular areas secures the diagnosis.

A slow upstroke to the carotid pulse indicates fixed obstruction to left ventricular emptying. This is the characteristic sign of aortic or subaortic stenosis. In supravalvular aortic stenosis the pulses in the upper part of the body may be asymmetric with the lesion causing propagation of a high velocity jet into the innominate artery. This results in bounding pulses in the carotid and brachial of that side. In contrast the left carotid and brachial are slow rising and more difficult to feel.

Collapsing or water hammer pulses are felt when the pulse pressure is widened by a low resistance run off from the systemic arterial system. Common causes include aortic regurgitation, persistent ductus arteriosus, aortopulmonary window and collateral arteries, truncus arteriosus or systemic arteriovenous fistula.

Blood pressure

This should be measured in both arms and a leg. This is mandatory if coarctation is suspected and should be repeated during exercise. It is important to use an appropriately sized cuff as spuriously high values will be recorded with a small or loosely fitting cuff. Doppler probes allow accurate estimation of the systolic pressure, especially when this is difficult to obtain by palpation or auscultation. Exaggeration of the normal tendency of the blood pressure to fall during inspiration (a paradoxical pulse) can accompany airway obstruction, congestive cardiac failure or pericardial tamponade.

Elevated blood pressure may be seen in coarctation (confined to the upper limbs), renal arterial stenosis or renal parenchymal disease. In many cases no specific cause can be found especially in the chronically cyanosed. Continuous ambulatory 24-hour recording devices will reveal the pattern of blood pressure variation over a complete day and can be useful in the assessment of suspected hypertension.

Jugular venous pulsation

The clinical assessment of the JVP will be familiar to all cardiologists. Graphical representation of the venous pulsation can be obtained with the use of a displacement transducer placed over the internal jugular.

Exaggerated 'a' waves imply increased resistance to right atrial emptying and occur in tricuspid stenosis, right ventricular hypertrophy, and after the Fontan procedure. The 'a' wave is not increased however when there is a coexisting ventricular septal defect as in Fallot's tetralogy and this is an important observation. A large 'a' wave may also be seen in conditions associated with left ventricular hypertrophy and episodic 'cannon' waves occur in cases of heart block when the atrium can contract against a closed tricuspid valve.

Prominence of the 'v' wave is characteristic of tricuspid regurgitation. In severe cases the venous wave form resembles a right ventricular pressure trace and neck pulsation is prominent. This is followed by a rapid 'y' descent except in cases of coexisting tricuspid stenosis when the right ventricular filling is delayed.

Precordial motion

Abnormal precordial motion may be seen or felt. Right ventricular over-activity causes a sustained systolic outward movement along the left sternal border (parasternal heave). This is most marked when there is both pressure and volume overload of the chamber. Interestingly, in Fallot's tetralogy this motion is brief and not prominent. This parallels the findings in examination of the venous pulses and is presumably due to the presence of the ventricular septal defect. An aneurysm of the right ventricular outflow tract (often the result of excessive resection of infundibular muscle or patching of the outflow tract during operative repair of Fallot's tetralogy) can cause a visible pulsatile motion at the mid and high left sternal edge. Rarely, abnormal pulsation of a dilated pulmonary artery may be felt in the region of the second left intercostal space. A palpable second sound should be sought when pulmonary hypertension is suspected.

The apical impulse usually represents activity of the left ventricle. This can be distorted in cases with a dilated right ventricle for example in atrial septal defect. A palpable presystolic outward movement at the apex may accompany a loud fourth heart sound in, for example, hypertrophic cardiomyopathy.

If a murmur is loud and includes certain low frequency vibrations it may be palpable as well as audible. Typical causes include non-rheumatic mitral regurgitation, pulmonary stenosis and ventricular septal defect. Additional information should then be sought by careful auscultation.

Auscultation of the heart

A systematic approach and a knowledge of the pathophysiology of congenital lesions can increase the diagnostic yield of auscultation.

The first heart sound coincides with the closure of the mitral and tricuspid valves. Although mitral and tricuspid components can be identified by phonocardiography they are usually heard as a single sound. Mitral closure is usually loudest and hence the first heart sound is maximal at the apex. Accentuation of the tricuspid component makes the sound louder at the left sternal border. This is noted in some cases of atrial septal defect.

A loud first heart sound is associated with conditions where the valve leaflets are widely separated as ventricular systole begins. For example, in patients with a short PR interval the blood flow caused by atrial systole keeps the leaflets open until ventricular systole forces them together. This rapid closure from a widely open position accentuates the first heart sound. Vigorous ventricular activity as in exercise, hyperthyroidism and hypertension can have the same effect. Late diastolic flow in mitral stenosis and in the increased right heart flow associated with atrial septal defects will respectively accentuate the mitral and tricuspid components of the first sound. Soft first heart sounds are a feature of poor myocardial contractility or a long PR interval.

The nature of the second sound must be clearly defined. Aortic and pulmonary components, if present, should be characterized and the effect of respiration on their splitting noted. If the components are separated by 20 ms or less they will appear single to the ear. Splitting of the second sound is usually best heard at the high or mid left sternal border. If splitting is most easily identified at the low left sternal border or apex then this may be due to the presence of a third heart sound or mitral opening artefact. Fixed or paradoxical splitting may be evident during quiet respiration but is best defined in held expiration. Normally the second sound is single for one or two beats, then splits more widely as systemic venous return gradually increases. With fixed splitting the sound is split at the start of held expiration and remains constant over the period of breath holding. With paradoxical splitting the split is present at the start of end expiration and becomes single over the next few beats.

A third heart sound is coincident with rapid early diastolic ventricular filling and is commonly heard in normal children and young adults. The gallop rhythm heard in young patients with congestive cardiac failure is either an accentuated third sound or a summation of third and fourth sounds as the associated tachycardia shortens diastole.

Additional sounds in early systole may have an aortic or pulmonary origin. Pulmonary ejection sounds can arise from a stenotic valve or a dilated pulmonary artery. The sound is maximal at the high left sternal border, is high pitched and generally louder in expiration. Aortic ejection sounds are often loudest at the apex and do not vary with respiration. Mid systolic clicks are most commonly associated with mitral valve prolapse and may be followed by a late apical systolic murmur. Both click and murmur may be intermittent.

Murmurs should be described in terms of timing, location, radiation, loudness, pitch and quality. Auscultation should be performed in the standard areas and also over the back, and at sites of any surgically created shunts or anastamoses. Changes in the murmur in relation to the respiratory cycle should be observed. Accurate timing of the murmur in relation to the heart sounds is vital. Cardiologists will be familiar with the more common systolic and diastolic murmurs. A murmur is said to be continuous if it extends through the second sound, even if it is not heard throughout the complete cardiac cycle. These occur in persistent ductus arteriosus when the murmur is best heard in the second left interspace. A patent shunt between a central systemic artery and a low pressure pulmonary artery (e.g. a Blalock anastamosis) will produce a continuous murmur best heard over the shunt. Other rare causes include arteriovenous fistulae, a significant arterial constriction and a ruptured aneurysm of the sinus of Valsalva. Continuous flow through the neck veins can give rise to a venous hum. This can be confused with the murmur of a patent ductus but is abolished if the patient lies flat or the ipsilateral neck veins are compressed.

2

Cross-sectional Echocardiography: Sequential Segmental Analysis

Introduction

There are two main 'languages' used for the description of congenital heart lesions. Both rely on a segmental approach, but have a different fundamental basis. Each has its supporters and detractors, but as with any language the most important thing is that those that use it understand its terms of reference. In this book we have chosen to use the sequential segmental analysis and definitions proposed by the Brompton Group since 1976; it is essentially based on the morbid anatomy of the heart but lends itself readily to cross-sectional echocardiographic determination.

In this chapter, we will describe how the segments of the heart, chamber morphology and relationships can be assessed using transthoracic cross-sectional echocardiography. In most adults, the only echocardiographic window that can provide detailed morphological information are the subcostal transverse abdominal sections, to show the abdominal great vessels, the apical four-chambered view and the parasternal long and short axis view. These are obviously the most familiar to physicians and cardiologists not primarily involved in the care of patients with congenital heart disease. For this reason, we will confine our comments to those features demonstrable in these simple views.

Transthoracic echocardiography – a segmental approach to cardiac diagnosis

Determination of atrial arrangement

The first segment of the heart to be determined is the atrial situs or atrial arrangement. The morphologically left and right atria each have their own

Table 1.   Atrial arrangement (determination of situs)

1. Usual (situs solitus)
2. Mirror image (situs inversus)
3. Right isomerism for left isomerism (bilateral/morphologically right or left atria)

specific features that allow their diagnosis independent of position. Their most consistent feature is the unique anatomy of the atrial appendages. The right atrial appendage is triangular and broad-based with extension of pectinate muscles around the atrioventricular groove. Conversely, the left atrial appendage is long and narrow with pectinate muscles confined to the appendage itself. Although it is now possible to demonstrate the atrial appendages in almost all cases by transoesophageal echo (see Chapter 3), this is rarely the case, even in small infants, with transthoracic echocardiography. We therefore have to rely on an indirect method.

The horizontal abdominal echocardiographic section at the level of the 10th or 11th thoracic vertebra (just beneath the sternal angle) will demonstrate clearly the relative position of aorta and inferior caval vein. There are four patterns of atrial arrangement (Table 1). In usual atrial arrangement, or situs solitus, there is normal arrangement of the abdominal great vessels with the aorta to the left of the spine and the inferior caval vein slightly anterior and to the right of the spine (Figure 1). In mirror image arrangement, the reverse is true. When there is right atrial isomerism the aorta and inferior caval vein are found on the same side of the

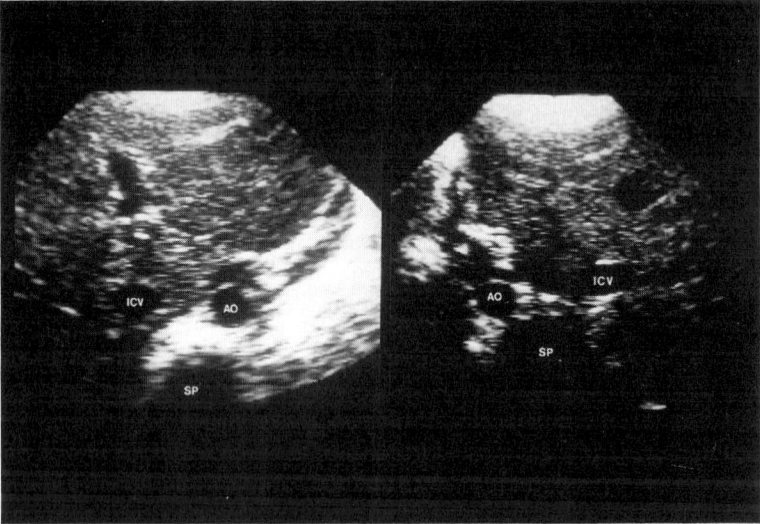

Figure 1.   Abdominal short axis views of the great vessels at the level of the 11th thoracic vertebra. Usual atria arrangement can be inferred (situs solitus) from the normal position of the aorta (AO) being to the left of the spine and inferior caval vein (ICV) on the right of the spine. In the right-hand panel, there is mirror image arrangement suggesting situs inversus.

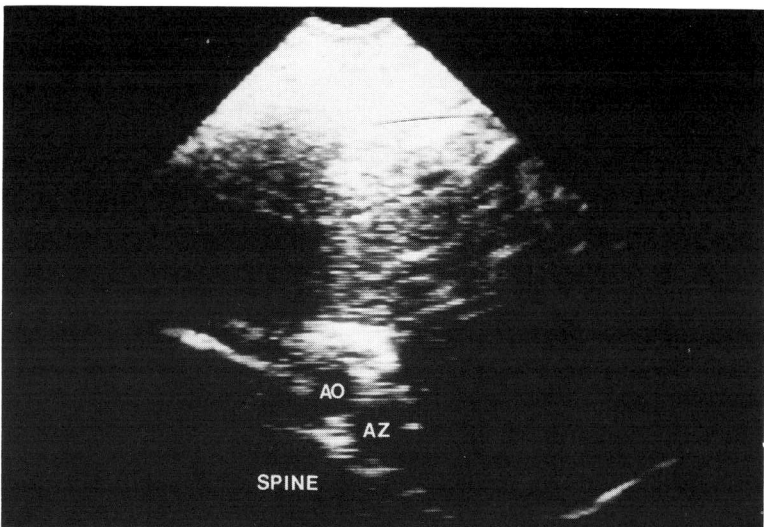

Figure 2.   Left atrial isomerism. This is inferred from the abdominal great vessels. The aorta is anterior and to the same side of the spine as the posterior azygus vein (AZ – see text for details).

spine, be it right or left, whereas with left atrial isomerism there is interruption of the inferior caval vein with a posterior azygous vein on the same side but posterior to the aorta in cross-section (Figure 2). As a consequence of interruption of the inferior caval vein, the hepatic veins drain directly to the atria.

Atrioventricular connection

Having defined the relative position of the morphologically right and left atriums, the atrioventricular connection can be established. Once again, there are several different types (Table 2).

The normal atrioventricular connection is, of course, biventricular and concordant: the morphologically right atrium is connected to the morphologically

Table 2.   Types of atrioventricular connection

Biventricular
   concordant
   discordant
   ambiguous (with atrial isomerism)

Univentricular
   double inlet
   absent right connection
   absent left connection

right ventricle and the left atrium is connected to the left ventricle no matter what their position. In discordant atrioventricular connection the right atrium connects to the left ventricle and vice versa. When there are two left or two right atria, then the connection can neither be concordant nor discordant and so it is described as ambiguous.

Which ventricle is which?

The atrioventricular connection can only be assigned once the morphology of the respective ventricle has been defined. There are several echocardiographic clues that one obtains from an apical four-chambered view that are helpful in this regard. Remember, the atrioventricular valve always goes with its respective ventricle. Definition of the morphology of the atrioventricular valves will there-fore define the morphology of the ventricle. The normal tricuspid valve is off-set with respect to the normal mitral valve, it being closer to the apex of the right ventricle than the mitral valve is to the apex of the left ventricle (Figure 3.) The offsetting is due to interposition of the atrioventricular septum, which separates the morphological left ventricle from the right atrium in the normal heart. There is therefore a problem in cases of inlet ventricular septal defects (where there is fibrous continuity of mitral and tricuspid valves) and in atrioventricular septal defects (where the atrioventricular septum is absent). Under these circumstances, we can rely on the chordal and tensor apparatus of the respective atrioventricular

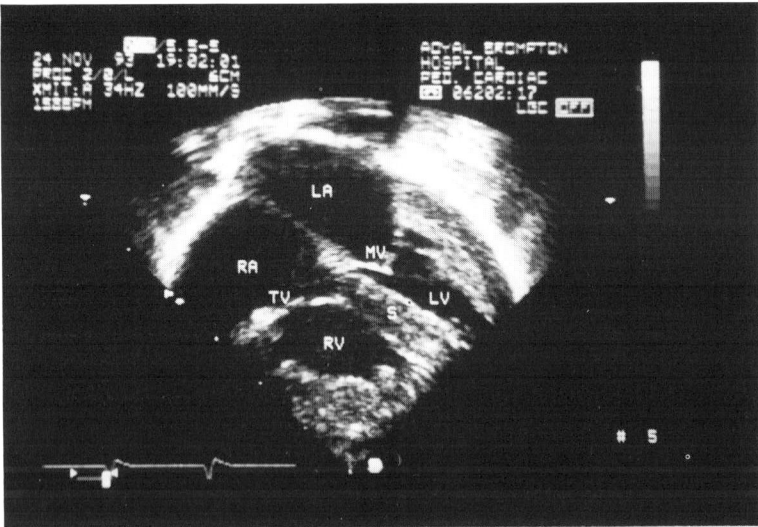

Figure 3.   The normal four-chamber projection. There is usual atrial arrangement. Note how the septal leaflet of the tricuspid valve is attached more distally on the septum than that of the mitral valve. Also, the mitral valve inserts into a lateral papillary muscle whereas the tricuspid valve has septal attachments. Thus there is a concordant atrioventricular connection (see text for details).

valves. The normal tricuspid valve has chordal attachments to the right side of the interventricular septum and to the right ventricular apex, whereas the mitral valve has chordal attachment to lateral papillary muscles, well away from the septum. The most consistent morphological abnormality is the apical trabecular pattern. In the right ventricle there are coarse apical trabeculations whereas in the left ventricle they are much finer. This is a difficult echocardiographic distinction but there is one feature of the apical trabecular pattern that allows differentiation. This is the moderator band, best seen in the apical four-chambered view and recognized as a transverse band of muscle towards the apex of the right ventricle. These definitions hold not only for the obviously biventricular heart where there are two well-formed ventricles each with its own inlet, trabecular, and outlet portions, but also when there is a univentricular atrioventricular connection. Univentricular atrioventricular connection will be described in detail in Chapter 10. The essential definition is that more than 75% of the existing atrioventricular mass connects to one or other of the ventricles. This is an arbitrary assignment. Thus in double inlet left ventricle, both atria connect predominantly to the left ventricle, there being a rudimentary and incomplete right ventricle. In absent right connection (also known as tricuspid atresia), the tricuspid valve is absent, there being an infolding of the floor of the right atrium and the roof of the rudimentary ventricle. The only exit from the right atrium is through the atrial septum, and the left atrium and its atrioventricular valve then usually connect to a dominant ventricle. Thus once again, the atrioventricular connection is univentricular. The differentiation of left from right ventricle under these circumstances cannot, of course, rely on the pattern of the atrioventricular junction or the morphology of the atrioventricular valves. Furthermore, it can be very difficult to differentiate the ventricles on the basis of their apical trabecular pattern. The rudimentary ventricle, be it a right or left ventricle, can be right or left sided, but a consistent feature is its anteroposterior relationship with the main chamber. If there is an anterior rudimentary ventricle, then it is almost certainly a right ventricle and if there is a posterior rudimentary ventricle then it is a left ventricle. This is obviously best seen in parasternal short and long axis projection. Just occasionally, no rudimentary chamber can be detected in these hearts. Under these circumstances, the connection is described as univentricular atrioventricular connection to an indeterminate ventricle.

Ventriculoarterial connection

Table 3.   Types of ventriculoarterial connection

1. Condordant
2. Discordant
3. Double outlet
4. Single outlet (infundibular pulmonary atresia, truncus arteriosus)

Having described the atrioventricular connection as well as the morphology and position of the ventricles, it should then be relatively straightforward to diagnose the ventriculoarterial connections. The aorta characteristically forms the aortic arch and gives rise to coronary arteries and head and neck vessels, whereas the pulmonary artery bifurcates. Although this statement is obvious, in practice it is sometimes rather difficult to display these typical features. In general, if there is a spiralling relationship of the great vessels, they will be normally related with the anterior vessel being the pulmonary artery (Figure 4). Conversely, if the great vessels appear to be parallel in parasternal long axis projection, the anterior vessel (be it left or right sided) will usually be the aorta (Figure 5). Having decided which vessel is which, it then needs to be assigned to its supporting ventricle. Here again an arbitrary decision is made. The 50–50 rule applies. If more than 50% of the diameter of the origin of the vessel is committed to a ventricle it is said to be connected to that ventricle. Thus double outlet right ventricle with subaortic ventricular septal defect may differ from tetralogy of Fallot only in the degree of aortic override that exists (it being more than 50% in double outlet, 50% or less in tetralogy of Fallot). All of these features, however, should be readily apparent from simple parasternal long axis views.

Other features

Clearly the other morphological variables in congenital heart disease are of equal importance to the basic segmental diagnosis. The connection of systemic and

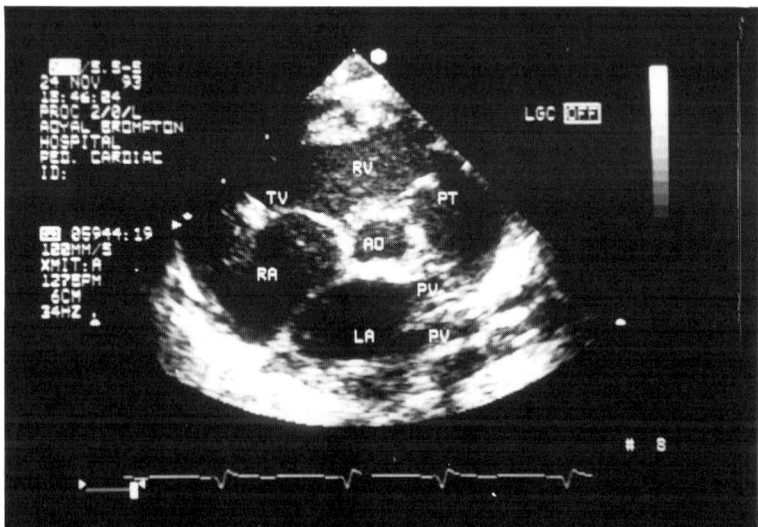

Figure 4. A normal parasternal short-axis view. Note the normal spiralling relationship of the great vessels. Under these circumstances the anterior great vessel is usually the pulmonary trunk.

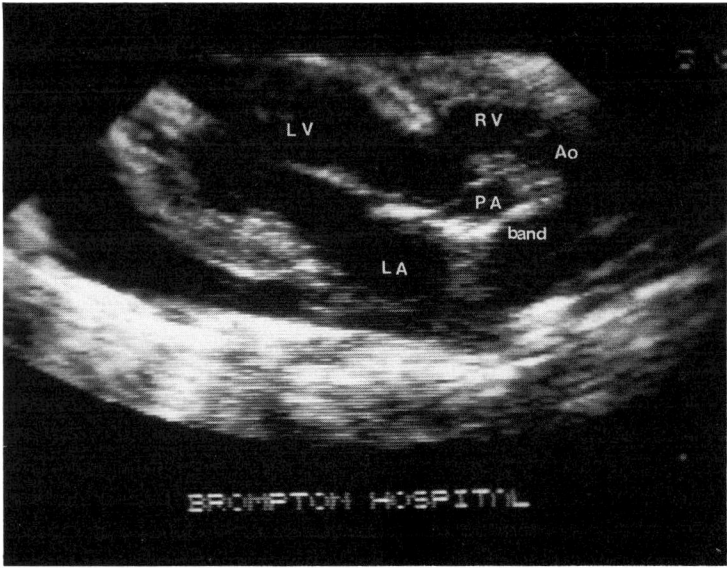

Figure 5. Double inlet left ventricle (LV) with a discordant ventriculoarterial connection. This shows several important features. The small rudimentary ventricle is anterior and is therefore a right ventricle (RV). There are parallel great vessels leaving the heart in long axis projection. Under these circumstances, the anterior vessel is usually the aorta (Ao). The ventriculoarterial connection is thus discordant. PA, pulmonary artery.

pulmonary veins, the presence or absence of intra-atrial and ventricular septal defects, the morphology of the atrioventricular valves and their tensor apparatus, as well as infundibular and valvar anatomy must all be examined and are discussed in more detail in other Chapters. In practice, some if not all of these features may be very difficult to display definitively in the adult with complex congenital heart disease. As with all imaging modalities, the failure to demonstrate something does not necessarily mean it is not there. Each case must be taken on its merits, but if there is any doubt then transoesophageal echo, magnetic resonance scanning or computed tomography will be required (see Chapters 3 and 5).

Doppler examination

By and large the principles of Doppler interrogation are similar to those used in adults with acquired heart disease. Clearly, probe positioning will vary, and to the non-specialist there is no substitute for duplex imaging with a steerable continuous wave facility. There are one or two caveats however. The modified Bernoulli equation is most accurate when defining gradients across a discrete stenosis. This is not always the case when there is congenital heart disease. There may be serious under-estimation of the peak instantaneous gradient when there is a long or complex stenosis (for example across an arterial duct, down a Blalock shunt, across the right ventricular outflow tract). Conversely, in high flow states, the apparent peak instantaneous gradient may be much higher than the peak-to-peak gradient assessed at cardiac catheterization. This is particularly the case when assessing a pulmonary arterial band for example. It is well known that the two measurements may be quite different in any case, but this difference is more marked in these conditions. This is almost certainly because the velocity proximal to the stenosis is elevated and so the measurement of a single maximal velocity is misleading when calculating the actual pressure gradient. Finally, the Doppler measurements cannot be taken in isolation. For example, a small gradient across a ventricular septal defect (implying a raised right ventricular pressure) cannot be used as evidence for pulmonary hypertension if right ventricular outflow tract obstruction has not been excluded.

Summary

Although the simplest investigation to do, transthoracic cross-sectional echo Doppler studies have the potential for being the most misleading. Only the individual operator knows his own limitations, but a realistic assessment must be taken into account when assessing the utility of any piece of information obtained in this way. None the less, using a stepwise and segmental approach to assessing all hearts, major mistakes in describing the basic anatomy should not be made. There is no place for guesswork however. If in doubt seek a specialist opinion before arranging potentially unnecessary additional tests.

Key references

McCartney FJ, Partridge JB, Shinebourne EA et al (1978) Identification of atrial situs. In Anderson RH and Shinebourne EA (eds) *Paediatric Cardiology*, pp. 16–26. Churchill Livingstone, Edinburgh.

Rigby ML, Redington AN (1989) Cross-sectional echocardiography. *Br Med Bull* **45**(4): 1036–60.

Shinebourne EA, McCartney RJ, Anderson RH (1976) Sequential chamber localisation – logical approach in diagnosis in congenital heart disease. *Br Heart J* **38**: 327–40.

3

Transoesophageal Echocardiography

In collaboration with SJD Brecker

Introduction

Over the past five years, transoesophageal echocardiography has developed into a highly sophisticated and versatile imaging technique, now integral to the diagnosis and management of congenital heart disease in adults. It has proved invaluable not only to the cardiologist for diagnosis, planning management and during interventional catheterization, but also to the anaesthetist and surgeon during the perioperative period and to the intensivist caring for the postoperative patient. Prior to any therapeutic intervention it is essential to define the complete sequential anatomical diagnosis and transoesophageal echocardiography may be the only way to clarify certain issues. During the perioperative and immediate postoperative period the technique is used to elevate ventricular function and surgical repair. It has become a gold standard for assessing vegetations and abscesses in infective endocarditis, prosthetic valve malfunction, intracardiac thrombus and aortic pathology (Figure 1). In the intensive care setting, transthoracic echocardiography is often difficult if not impossible, particularly in adults with congenital heart disease in whom chest drains, wound dressings and ventilation may make transthoracic images uninterpretable. Transoesophageal echocardiography is conventionally performed at the bedside in such patients, and provides information unobtainable in any other way.

Technical aspects

Original transoesophageal probes were developed in the late 1970s and early 1980s and were bulky, with limited capability. Single-plane two-dimensional scanning was developed in the 1980s with a 5 MHz transducer mounted at the tip of a flexible and steerable endoscope. In the last five years there have been rapid technological advances with reduction in size of the transducer and probe

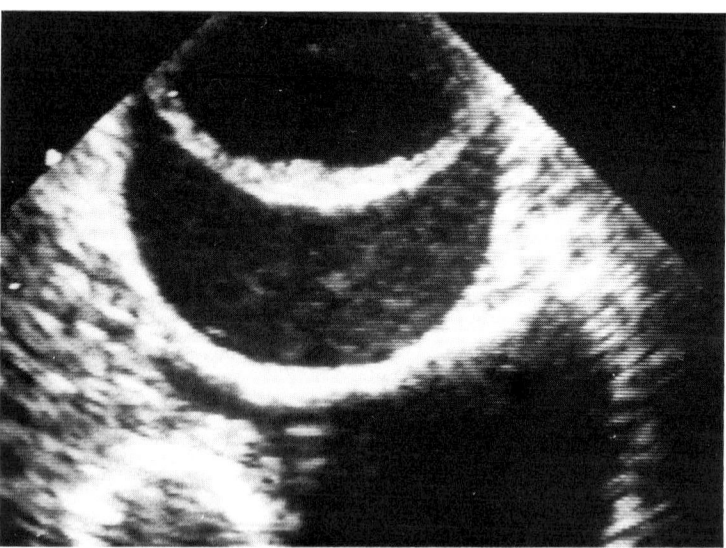

Figure 1.   Aortic dissection in a Marfan patient. Transverse plane transoesophageal echocardiogram of the descending aorta from a patient with Marfan's syndrome. Note the intimal flap, and spontaneous contrast signifying sluggish flow in the false lumen.

width, increase in the number of elements so improving image quality, and addition of biplane and multiplane imaging. In addition, pulsed wave Doppler, continuous wave and colour flow Doppler are now integral in all probes. Biplane systems utilize two phased-array transducers mounted next to one another, and multiplane systems have an electrically or mechanically steered transducer of either the phased-array or mechanical type. Reduction in overall size of the transducer has extended the applications to paediatric and neonatal patients. The latest technological advances are aimed at developing three-dimensional images of the heart in motion, and systems are already commercially available. At present the computer-based image processing for three-dimensional studies is cumbersome and resolution is not high, but these aspects will undoubtedly improve.

The clinical role of transoesophageal echocardiography ———

The indications and clinical applications of transoesophageal echocardiography are summarized in Tables 1 and 2, and will be discussed in greater detail later. Transoesophageal echocardiography is not a substitute for a careful transthoracic study; the information provided by transoesophageal echocardiography must be regarded as complementary, and the two methods can be regarded as synergistic. An abnormality may be suspected from a transthoracic study and confirmed on

Table 1. Indications for transoesophageal echocardiography in adult congenital heart disease

Complete sequential anatomical diagnosis
Infective endocarditis of the native and prosthetic valve
    Vegetation
    Abscess
Native and prosthetic valve function
    Stenosis
    Regurgitation
Atrial and atrial septal abnormalities
Pulmonary venous anomalies
    Drainage
    Obstruction
Conduit, shunt and baffle function
Pericardial effusion
Ventricular function
Intracardiac source of embolism
Aortic disease
    Dissection and rupture
    Aneurysmal dilatation

Table 2. Applications of transoesophageal echocardiography in adult congenital heart disease

Catheter laboratory
    Diagnosis
    Interventional procedures, e.g. device closure of atrial septal defect, balloon dilatation of stenosed
    valves or baffles, etc.
Operating theatre
    Diagnosis confirmed and refined
    Haemodynamic monitoring and fluid management
    Monitoring ventricular function
    Assessment of surgical repair – valve competence/residual septal defect, etc.
Intensive care unit
    Ventricular function
    Prosthetic valve function
    Postoperative competence of valve repair/septal defect closure
    Pericardial effusion and tamponade
    Endocarditis – vegetation and abscess

transoesophageal echocardiography, whilst areas of the heart blind from the oesophagus (such as the left ventricular outflow tract in a patient with a mechanical prosthesis in the mitral position) may be clearly seen from the thorax. Nevertheless transoesophageal echocardiography has a number of advantages over the transthoracic approach, including proximity to the heart without interposition of lung and bone, a greater signal-to-noise ratio and higher transducer frequency improving image quality, and that certain structures in adults such as the atrial appendages may only be imaged from the oesophagus. Furthermore, transoesophageal echocardiography has proved invaluable in the operating theatre, catheter laboratory and intensive care unit, when other imaging modalities may be impractical to use or fail to provide adequate information. The diagnostic information obtained from any imaging modality with high sensitivity must however be used in the appropriate clinical context. Thus it is important to remember that a small mobile mass on a prosthetic valve has more significance in a febrile patient with positive blood cultures than one without such clinical features. The clinical usefulness of the technique may be increased if there is a clear question to be answered which should be defined prior to the study.

How to set up a 'TOE' lab

For general outpatient work, the ideal arrangement is to have a purpose-designed and dedicated area for transoesophageal echocardiography. In a number of centres sessions are arranged in endoscopy suites, and this may be a suitable alternative. In any event, the room must be of sufficient size to allow comfortable accommodation of the patient, operator, assistants and equipment. Oxygen and suction must be available, together with monitoring equipment including a pulse oximeter. Full resuscitation equipment must be nearby. Ideally, cabinets should be available in the room to store the probe and all ancillary equipment such as intravenous cannulae, syringes, local anaesthetic spray and gel, mouth guards, video tapes, etc. Facilities for cleaning the probe should be available; on completion of a study the probe should be washed with a dilute antiseptic soap solution, rinsed and placed in a glutaraldehyde solution for 15 minutes. Following this the probe should be rinsed thoroughly, dried and stored. The use of sheaths varies between units, but if this is done then care must be taken to ensure that ultrasound gel is placed at the tip of the sheath next to the transducer to ensure good image quality. Local arrangements will determine who assists the cardiologist performing the study; this may be a cardiac technician or nurse, but ideally two assistants should be available – one to care for the patient during the study and the other to alter settings on the ultrasound machine.

How to perform a transoesophageal electrocardiogram

Patients should be prepared for the procedure in an identical fashion to those undergoing upper gastrointestinal endoscopy, and a four- to six-hour fast is required. The patient should first of all have a clear understanding of why a transoesophageal echocardiogram is required, and why the oesophageal approach is necessary. Patients with gastrointestinal disease often expect such a test, those with heart disease do not. We believe that the most important factor determining patient cooperation is a sensitive and thorough explanation of the sensations that the patient will experience throughout the procedure. Reassurance is given that the test is not dangerous nor painful, nor does it interfere with normal breathing. The discomfort of the probe passing the pharynx is described, and patients are told that it does not last long, and once the probe is in the oesophagus it becomes much more tolerable. Patients are told the likely length of the procedure, asked to confirm that they have had nothing to eat or drink for at least four hours prior to the procedure, and finally asked for informed consent. Those under the age of sixteen will also need their parents' consent. Note is made of any dental caps or crowns, and dentures are removed. A local anaesthetic spray (Xylocaine) is given to the pharynx whilst the patient is sitting up. Patients are then instructed to lie on their left-hand side, with their right knee flexed and placed in front of the left leg, with arms by the side. The head is comfortably flexed, and suction is provided to clear any oral secretions.

This brings us to the question of sedation. Older patients tolerate the procedure far better than the young, and sedation should be used for all adolescents and young adults. A proportion of patients over the age of 40 may not require sedation, and in our unit are given this option. A short-acting benzodiazepine such as midazolam (Hypnovel) is the most appropriate single agent, but dose titration is critical. 1–2 mg aliquots are given until the patient is only just able to obey commands. Very careful consideration to respiration should be given before exceeding 10 mg, and the benzodiazepine antagonist flumazenil (Anexate) should be available. Addition of a small dose of an opiate such as fentanyl 50, 100 µg, may be advantageous in certain patients, but once again attention to respiratory function is important. In patients with suspected aortic dissection, a formal protocol should be established involving adequate premedication and procedural sedation, and hypotensive agents such as labetalol should be infused to maintain the systolic blood pressure below 100 mmHg. Probe insertion in the inadequately sedated patient can lead to elevation of the blood pressure by 20–30 mmHg which is clearly undesirable in such patients. At present it is our practice not to administer intravenous antibiotics, even to those with complex congenital heart disease as current evidence suggests that it is unnecessary.

Once the patient has had topical anaesthesia and is adequately sedated in the left lateral position, the probe can be inserted using one of two techniques. The operator places his left index and middle fingers into the oropharynx to act as a guide, and with his right hand advances the probe into the oesophagus asking the patient to swallow as he does so. The probe should be lubricated with a 2% lignocaine gel. Once the probe is in place, a plastic bite guard is positioned between the teeth. The alternative method which is suitable for smaller patients, is to place the bite guard between the teeth initially, and to pass the lubricated probe into the oropharynx. The patient is instructed to swallow, and the probe advanced into the oesophagus. Introduction of the probe into an anaesthetized and ventilated patient is different. The patient will be on their back, and the head should be in the midline and slightly flexed. The endotracheal tube can be gently placed to one side of the mouth, but care must be taken not to displace it. The probe can usually be placed in the oesophagus blindly by directing the tip to the back of the pharynx behind the endotracheal tube, and advancing gently until images of the heart are obtained. The probe should not be advanced against resistance and direct vision using a laryngoscope may be required. Manipulation of the probe can only be learnt by practical experience, and for a comprehensive description of all horizontal, vertical and intermediate scan planes the reader is directed to the bibliography at the end of this chapter. The probe may be advanced and withdrawn, rotated along its long axis, and deflected in the anteroposterior and lateral planes. Exact positioning is guided by the two-dimensional image, but manipulation to obtain standard views will vary between individual patients based upon variations in the cardiac position and rotation. Nevertheless, a stepwise and logical approach to obtaining the views in each plane should be followed.

Contraindications and complications

Oesophageal pathology is a relative if not absolute contraindication to the procedure, and strictures or varices preclude the investigation. In those with congenital heart disease the presence of vascular rings or previous oesophageal surgery are relative contraindications. Inability to obtain images occurs in 1–5% of studies due to patient intolerance, and if the procedure is critical to management decisions, then consideration should be given to performing the procedure under general anaesthetic. Complications are rare but include cardiac arrhythmias including ectopic beats, atrial fibrillation, ventricular tachycardia and even complete heart block. Oesophageal perforation occurs in less than 0.01%. Bacterial endocarditis and death have been reported anecdotally, but are extremely rare.

Indications and applications

Rather than listing all possible reasons for performing a transoesophageal study, this section is designed to give the reader an overview of the more common roles of the technique. Tables 1 and 2 summarize the main indications and applications of transoesophageal echocardiography.

Complete sequential anatomical diagnosis

Transoesophageal echocardiography may be the only way to complete a sequential anatomical diagnosis in an adult with complex congenital heart disease. Surgical procedures and shunts may have been performed years before without

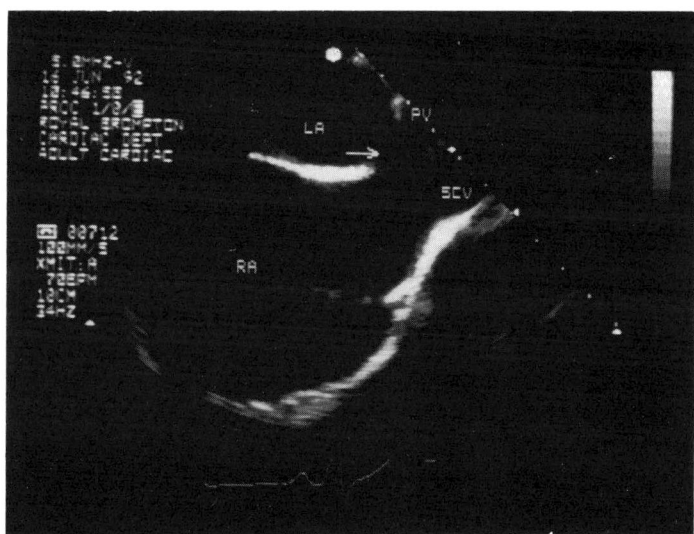

Figure 2. Superior sinus venosus atrial septal defect. Longitudinal plane transoesophageal echocardiogram showing the sinus venosus atrial septal defect or the 'superior vena cava defect'. Note the defect is in the upper part of the interatrial septum (arrowed), causing the superior vena cava to override the septum. LA, left atrium; PV, pulmonary valve; RA, right atrium; SCV, superior caval vein.

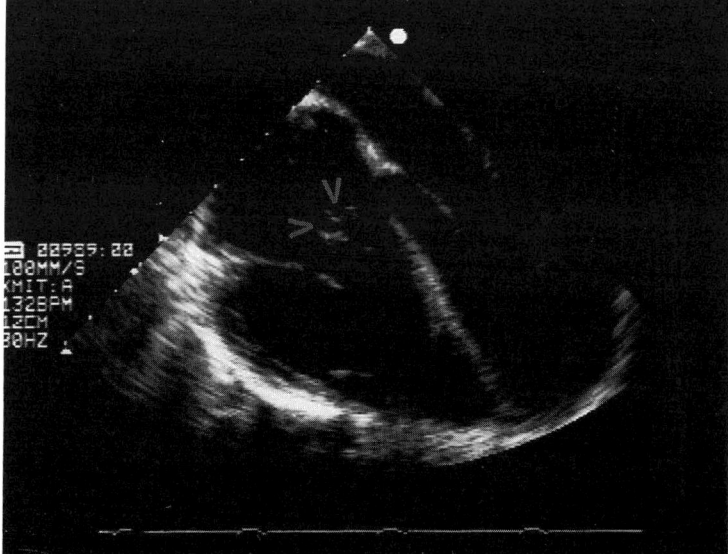

Figure 3. Ruptured sinus of Valsalva aneurysm. Transverse plane transoesophageal echocardiogram showing a four-chamber view. Note the ring shadow in the right atrium which was a ruptured sinus of Valsalva aneurysm of the windsock type. Note also the dilated right-sided chambers.

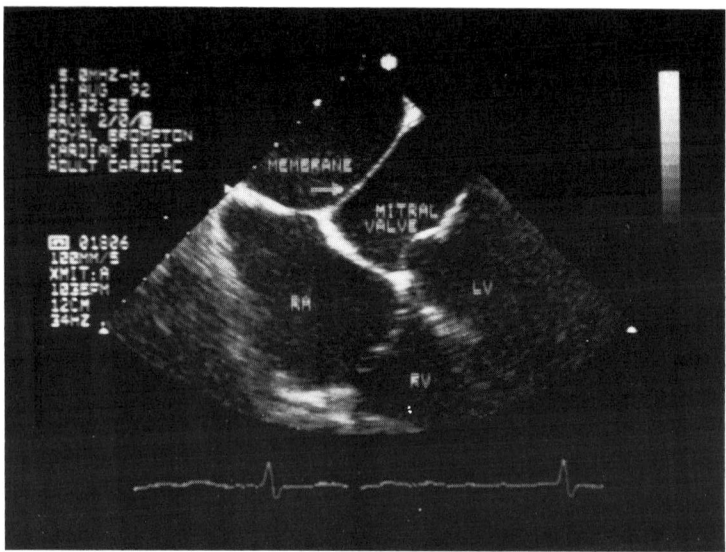

Figure 4. Cor triatriatum. Transverse plane transoesophageal echocardiogram showing a clear membrane in the left atrium dividing it into a proximal pulmonary venous chamber, and a distal chamber in communication with the mitral orifice. LV, left ventricle; RA, right atrium; RV, right ventricle.

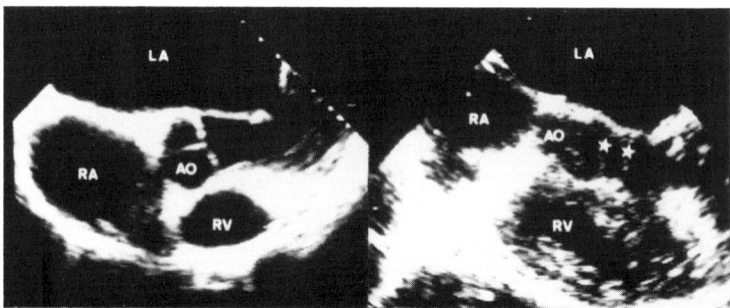

Figure 5. Subaortic stenosis. Vertical plane transoesophageal echocardiograms showing the left ventricular outflow tract with fibromuscular subaortic stenosis (left hand panel) and normal appearances (right hand panel) for comparison. There are two ridges due to a spiralling ridge seen (stars).

a complete anatomical diagnosis, and full details of the surgical findings and procedures may not be available. Atrial situs is clarified with excellent imaging of appendage anatomy, the whole of the interatrial septum can be imaged (Figure 2) and the atrioventricular connection is often refined with clear definition of chordal insertion, straddling and override. Interatrial abnormalities including fistulous connections (Figure 3) and membranes (Figure 4) may be clearly identified. Rudimentary ventricular chambers can be identified and the ventricular morphology and ventriculoarterial connections elucidated. Biplane and multiplane images give exceptional anatomical definition of the outflow tracts

(Figure 5) and the origin and structure of the great vessels. All four pulmonary veins can usually be identified and abnormalities of site and character of drainage can be determined. Finally, associated anomalies such as a patent ductus arteriosus or aortic coarctation may be identified, and the function of extra-cardiac structures such as conduits and shunts may be assessed.

Infective endocarditis

Vegetations may be seen on both native and prosthetic valves with a high degree of resolution (1 mm versus 3 mm for transthoracic echocardiography). Abscess cavities may be defined in regions of the heart normally difficult to image from the transthoracic approach, such as the posterior aortic root behind a prosthetic aortic valve. Defining the anatomy of the abscess may assist the surgeon in planning the operative approach. Paraprosthetic regurgitant jets to the side of a mitral prosthesis may be eccentric and difficult to characterize by any other technique. Leaflet perforation, valve dehiscence and fistulous connections can all be imaged with a high degree of resolution. It is important to realize that a negative study does not exclude the diagnosis, and shadowing of areas behind prosthetic valves remains as much of a problem to the oesophageal approach as that from the front.

Native and prosthetic valve function

Transoesophageal echocardiography must only be used as an adjunct to trans-thoracic echocardiography and Doppler in assessing valvular function. The M-mode echocardiogram of the left ventricular cavity provides a wealth of information which should not be discarded in favour of new technology. Never-theless the oesophageal approach is excellent for assessing forward mitral gradients, and for detecting eccentric jets of mitral regurgitation. The submitral apparatus can be assessed with regard to suitability for balloon valvuloplasty. The aortic valve cusps may be imaged with spectacular clarity, particularly using intermediate scan planes.

Atrial and atrial septal abnormalities

Both atria and appendages are particularly well-imaged from the oesophageal approach, and septal defects may be clearly defined. Transoesophageal echocar-diography has become essential in the assessment of suitability of atrial septal defects for device closure. Sinus venosus defects, often difficult to image from transthoracic echocardiography may be defined particularly well from long axis scan planes (Figure 2). Associated anomalies of pulmonary venous drainage may also be confirmed.

Pulmonary venous abnormalities

All four pulmonary veins can usually be identified draining to the left atrium using biplane scanning, although the right lower vein can be difficult to demonstrate selectively. Anomalous drainage is often well demonstrated, with imaging of a pulmonary venous confluence. Pulsed Doppler recordings are easy to obtain from within the pulmonary veins, and equally easy to over-interpret. The factors determining pulmonary venous flow are multiple and complex, and will not be discussed further.

Conduit, shunt and baffle function

Extracardiac conduits are extremely difficult to image from the transthoracic approach, particularly in young adults. They are often anterior and run vertically. Longitudinal plane transoesophageal imaging may often demonstrate the entire length of the conduit, and together with Doppler, sites of stenosis may be assessed. Conduit regurgitation and function of the conduit valve may be similarly evaluated. Transoesophageal echocardiography provides clear views of both the systemic and pulmonary venous limbs of baffle reconstructions for transposition of the great arteries. Pulmonary venous baffle obstruction and obstruction to superior or inferior vena caval flow into the systemic venous baffle may be demonstrated. Cavopulmonary anastomoses may sometimes be seen, and this is best done in the longitudinal plane. Atriopulmonary connections such as the Fontan procedure are easier to assess, and their flow characteristics determined with pulsed Doppler.

Aortic disease

Transoesophageal echocardiography has, in a number of units, become the imaging modality of choice for defining aortic disease, whether it be aneurysmal dilatation or dissection (Figure 1). It is ideal in the patient with suspected dissection, as it can be performed in the intensive care unit. Additional details of the dissection may be determined, including extent, entry and exit sites and involvement of coronary arteries and head and neck vessels. A small length of the upper ascending and proximal transverse aorta is however blind to transoesophageal echocardiography due to interposition of the trachea.

Assessment of surgical repair

Transoesophageal echocardiography can contribute to perioperative management of almost any surgical repair for congenital heart disease. In addition to simple assessment of the operative procedure, monitoring of ventricular function and fluid balance can assist the anaesthetist. Repair of septal defects, conduit construction, valve repair and resection of for example infundibular obstruction may all be evaluated, and immediate action may be taken by the surgeon if the result is unsatisfactory.

Summary

When transoesophageal echocardiography was first introduced into clinical practice, its values, roles and benefits were undefined. Now it is indispensable to cardiologists, cardiac surgeons and anaesthetists, particularly those caring for adults with congenital heart disease. The indications, advantages and pitfalls are increasingly recognized as the method has become more widely used, and modern management of adult congenital heart disease would be deficient without it.

Key references

Fisher EA, Stahl JA, Budd JH, Goldman ME (1991) Transesophageal echocardiography: Procedures and clinical application. *J Am Coll Cardiol* **18**: 1333–48.

Seward JB, Khandheria BK, Oh JK et al (1988) Transesophageal echocardiography: Technique, anatomic correlations, implementation, and clinical applications. *Mayo Clin Proc* **63**: 649–80.

Seward JB, Khandheria BK, Edwards WD et al (1990) Biplanar transesophageal echocardiography: Anatomic correlations, image orientation and clinical applications. *Mayo Clin Proc* **65**: 1193–213.

Seward JB, Khandheria BK, Oh JK, Freeman WK, Tajik AJ (1992) Critical appraisal of transesophageal echocardiography: Limitations, pitfalls, and complications. *J Am Soc Echocardiogr* **5**: 288–305.

Stümper O, Fraser AG, Ho SY et al (1990) Transesophageal echocardiography in the longitudinal axis: correlation between anatomy and images and its clinical implications. *Br Heart J* **64**: 282–88.

Weintraub R, Shiota T, Elkadi T et al (1992) Transesophageal echocardiography in infants and children with congenital heart disease. *Circulation* **86**: 711–22.

4 Dynamic Exercise Testing

In collaboration with Dr S Cullen

Introduction

Dynamic testing of cardiovascular haemodynamics forms part of the assessment of the grown-up patient with congenital heart disease. Although many data can be derived from cardiac evaluation at rest, it is how the cardiovascular system responds to stress and the demands of exercise that may be most important. In addition to the physiological data obtained, the psychological reassurance to patient and doctor may be equally valuable. Sometimes the results are surprisingly good, and sometimes surprisingly bad. Right-sided disease tends to be remarkably well tolerated, whereas exercise capacity may be markedly limited by systemic ventricular dysfunction which may appear mild to moderate when measured at rest. Interpretation of physiological data obtained during dynamic testing is critical and must be compared both to normal data obtained in the individual testing centre and to that expected for the lesion. All patients have reduced exercise capacity after the Fontan procedure, for example, and relative performance (to others and in the individual during follow-up) is clearly more important.

Whereas exercise is part of normal life and socialization in children, it must be remembered that in adolescence and adults, the ability to exercise is mainly determined by desire and habit. Thus, exercise intolerance due to lack of conditioning is a normal finding even in populations without congenital heart disease and this should be borne in mind.

The mode of investigation used will depend on the particular question which is being addressed. Thus if a transvalvar gradient is the issue, Doppler echocardiographic measurement of peak instantaneous gradient during exercise or drug-induced tachycardia, e.g. isoprenaline/dobutamine infusion could be used. Alternatively, testing at the time of cardiac catheterization may be employed. Similar methods are useful if the restrictive nature of a ventricular septal defect needs to be defined, e.g. in the case of double inlet left ventricle with ventriculoarterial discordance.

In most centres treadmill exercise testing with monitoring of blood pressure, heart rate, oxygen saturation and electrocardiograph is routinely employed. These tests can be supplemented with cross-sectional and Doppler echocardiographic examination during exercise. More detailed investigation of the cardiorespiratory response to exercise can be undertaken in specialized laboratories. Thus measurement of mixed expired gases by re-breathing techniques using respiratory mass-spectrometry may be used to establish cardiac output response and anaerobic threshold during testing and maximum effort performance but are largely research tools at present.

Exercise parameters

Respiratory gas exchange

Several methods are available for measurement of metabolic gas exchange from which oxygen consumption (VO_2), carbon dioxide production (VCO_2), and minute ventilation can be calculated both at rest and during exercise. The anaerobic threshold, variously defined, has been used as one index of cardiorespiratory adaptation to physiological stress and exercise. Originally, the Douglas bag was employed for the collection of all gases expired during a given period of time. The Douglas bag was analysed for oxygen content and volume and it was then possible to calculate the oxygen consumption during the period of collection. The modern respiratory mass spectrometers and pneumotachygraphs have greatly simplified the collection of these data. It is now possible to calculate the above parameters during a single breath. While breathing room air, all the expired gases from the patient are passed via a Hans Rudolf one-way valve through a pneumotachygraph which calculates the volume of flow. The capillary inlet portion of the respiratory mass spectrometer is placed at this point and one can accurately determine the amount of expired oxygen and carbon dioxide. The use of an on-line microcomputer allows easy management of data collection and continuous calculation of oxygen consumption, carbon dioxide production and minute ventilation on a breath-by-breath basis.

When measurements of respiratory gas exchange are combined with treadmill testing or bicycle ergometry, detailed information on cardiorespiratory responses to physiological stress and exercise can be derived. Delivery of blood to the tissues by the heart dictates the maximum oxygen uptake. The better conditioned or highly trained the individual the higher the oxygen consumption levels which can be obtained. A plateau of oxygen consumption occurs at higher levels of work and at this point carbon dioxide production increases as the patient exercises anaerobically (anaerobic threshold).

Most of these detailed studies are reserved for research purposes, and even then serial measurements over a period of time are more important than individual observations. They may be particularly important in those conditions in which heart–lung interactions play an important part in determining the cardiac output, e.g. following a Fontan operation or its modifications. In other conditions they have only limited relevance to our individual patient's clinical status.

Doppler echocardiography

Doppler echocardiographic measurements of peak-to-peak instantaneous trans-valvar gradients are more easily performed in patients exercising in the supine position, although it is well documented that the responses to supine exercise are different to those performed in the upright position. Other than assessment of transvalvar and/or outflow tract gradients during exercise, there are really no other routine clinical indications for Doppler echocardiography in dynamic testing in grown-up patients with congenital heart disease. In some conditions, such as aortic valve stenosis this technique has been used to assess timing of surgical or transcatheter intervention. However, there are practical limitations to the use of Doppler echocardiography during upright exercise, not least maintaining contact between probe and the patient's chest.

ST segment change

Ischaemic heart disease is the primary indication for exercise testing in adults. Many studies have documented a correlation between changes of the ST segment of the electrocardiogram and the presence of coronary artery disease. Patients with congenital heart defects frequently have right bundle branch block and abnormalities of ventricular repolarization on their standard 12-lead electrocar-diogram either related to the underlying defect or following surgical intervention. This makes interpretation of changes in ST segments extremely difficult and imprecise. One possible exception is isolated unoperated valvar aortic stenosis where significant ST changes occuring with exercise, indicate some degree of myocardial ischaemia.

Arrhythmia

This is a difficult area. Most 'arrhythmias' on exercise turn out to be sinus tachycardia and this knowledge alone can be reassuring to both patient and doctor. If a clinically important arrhythmia is manifest reproducibly on exercise then testing to assess the effects of treatment may rarely be useful. The problem comes when there is failure to reproduce symptoms during monitored exercise. Unfortunately this tends to be the most common scenario, and under these circumstances it may be more appropriate to undertake more overtly provocative testing during electrophysiological study.

What to expect from patients with congenital heart disease —

Left-to-right shunts (operated/unoperated)

The majority of patients with significant left-to-right shunts seen by the adult physician will already have undergone surgical intervention. Assuming the absence of pulmonary hypertension one would expect normal data from exercise testing allowing for the level of the patient's conditioning. The more significant the residual shunt, the greater the reduction in exercise tolerance.

Patients with established pulmonary hypertension, either primary or secondary, have reduced exercise tolerance and are at risk of ventricular arrhythmias during exercise. The value of exercise testing in these patients is limited other than perhaps to corroborate the patients' symptoms. As with all forms of exercise testing full resuscitation equipment must be available during the exercise test and the presence of an experienced physician and nurse is required.

Valvar stenosis

Patients with pulmonary valvar stenosis usually have a normal exercise tolerance. If the transvalvar Doppler gradient is measured during exercise it will increase as the cardiac output rises. Exercise-induced peak instantaneous gradients above 100 mmHg are considered by most as an indication for intervention. It is clearly a matter of personal preference but we feel that such exercise data adds little to that obtainable at rest, and so rarely use exercise testing to guide clinical decision-making.

Coarctation of the aorta

It is pointless performing exercise evaluation in patients with existing coarctation of the aorta, as the obstruction needs to be relieved whatever the result. More important is the assessment of blood pressure response after repair (particularly if performed late). This should be a routine part of postoperative evaluation as a subset of patients have dangerous elevation of blood pressure on exercise and require antihypertensive therapy even if normotensive at rest.

Cyanotic heart defects

Tetralogy of Fallot

Following successful correction of tetralogy of Fallot most patients have a good quality of life and reasonable exercise tolerance. The association between residual

pulmonary regurgitation and reduced exercise tolerance has recently been documented. Simply stated, the more severe the pulmonary regurgitation, the more
marked is the reduction in the exercise tolerance. Ventricular arrhythmias which
are known to occur in a high proportion of survivors of surgery of tetralogy of
Fallot may be detected on routine exercise testing. If associated with symptoms,
they should be treated aggressively.

Intra-atrial repair for complete transposition of the great arteries

Subclinical venous pathway obstruction following Mustard's Senning operation
for transposition of the great arteries may be revealed on exercise testing and can
be responsible for reduced exercise tolerance in these patients. Pulse Doppler
echocardiographic examination of the systemic and pulmonary venous pathways
will detect the obstruction in most cases but all probably require further
investigation with cardiac catheterization and angiography. When compared to
the normal population, maximal exercise tolerance is reduced in this group of
patients. Submaximal exercise capacity is usually normal, however, and this best
relates to daily activities. Another important use of exercise testing in these
patients is the demonstration of rhythm during exercise. Although resting nodal
rhythm is common, sinus rhythm is usually promptly restored on minimal
exertion.

Fontan operation

The Fontan operation or its modifications is widely used in those congenital
heart defects in which biventricular repair is impossible. As a rule, exercise
ability is reduced in this group and is approximately 50–70% of that achieved
by a normal population. This is presumably related to a limited ability to
increase cardiac output with increasing heart rate and the complex interraction
between heart and lungs in these patients is currently being studied. Serial
studies from the Mayo Clinic have shown that there should be little deterioration during the first decade following the procedure, and if demonstrated this
is itself an indication for careful reevaluation of the Fontan circuit in these
patients.

Summary

Although widely used, the role of exercise testing in adult patients with congenital heart defects remains to be precisely defined. It may prove useful for
corroboration of patients' symptoms and to monitor the progression of disease
and/or benefits of medical or surgical intervention. Each case must be taken on
its merits and the results assessed appropriately.

Key references

Bowyer JJ, Burst C, Till JA, Lincoln C, Shinebourne EA (1990) Exercise ability after Mustards operation. *Arch Dis Child* **65**: 865–70.

Carvalho JS, Shinebourne EA, Busst C, Rigby ML, Redington AN (1992) Exercise capacity after complete repair of tetralogy of Fallot: Deleterious effects of residual pulmonary regurgitation. *Br Heart J* **67**: 470–73.

Nir A, Driscoll DJ, Mottram CD *et al.* (1993) Cardiorespiratory response to exercise after the Fontan operation: a serial study. *J Am Coll Cardiol* **22**: 216–20.

5 Magnetic Resonance Imaging and Computed Tomography

In collaboration with Dr S Kaddoura

Introduction

Cross-sectional (both transthoracic and transoesophageal) echo Doppler studies can usually provide excellent high quality anatomical and functional information (see Chapters 2 and 3). Although still limited to use in some specialized centres, magnetic resonance imaging (MRI) and ultrafast cine computed tomography (CT), have also progressed and are now a useful adjunct, rather than an alternative, to echo Doppler. Most cardiologists now have access to one or other, but when evaluating the utility of these new techniques, it is important to compare them with the existing modalities.

The beauty of MRI and ultrafast CT techniques is that they can potentially provide, in a single study lasting approximately one hour, information regarding:

1. The anatomy of the heart and great vessels, and their connections.
2. Valvular and cardiac chamber function.
3. The haemodynamics of blood flow, including shunt estimation, and, in the case of MRI, of pressure.
4. Pre- and postoperative evaluation of patients with complex cardiac lesions.

Just as with everything else in this book, experience of the problems is a prerequisite to success. It is unfair to expect a radiologist with no experience of congenital heart disease correctly to interpret a CT or MRI scan in a patient with complex heart disease. In the right hands, however, these techniques come into their own.

The development of rapid-scanning techniques coupled with electrocardiographic triggering to overcome the problem of cardiac motion have made CT and MRI techniques of great use in adults with congenital heart disease. High-quality three-dimensional images can be produced in a number of planes (e.g. sagittal, coronal, transverse, left anterior oblique, etc., and combinations of these), some of which are not possible with echo Doppler.

Computed tomography

Conventional CT scanning was limited for use in cardiac disease by the low temporal resolution due to the long data acquisition times needed, leading to serious motion artefacts. A major step forward came with the development of ultrafast cine CT scanners (such as the Imatron C-100 Ultrafast CT, Imatron, San Francisco, California, USA) which allow the collection of multislice, rapid acquisition data.

An electron beam is fired from a gun and swept at the speed of light across four tungsten targets located beneath the patient. Each target produces two fans of X-rays which pass through the subject and are detected by a semicircular array of X-ray detectors above the patient. The entire heart and great vessels can be scanned in 3D, and in each 50 ms interval, two side-by-side 8 mm thick tomograms are produced. Electrocardiographic triggering and intravenous contrast are used.

There are three main ultrafast CT scanning modes, each providing a different type of information:

1. Flow mode

This is probably the most important mode and gives information regarding:

○ cardiac output;
○ shunt size;
○ anatomical detail, such as of the pulmonary veins, by using subtraction techniques in the venous phase.

2. Cine mode

The CT scanner is fired as rapidly as possible, giving sequential images of a single heartbeat at 50 ms intervals. A closed loop of images can be played through in real time. The endocardial and epicardial surfaces can be easily identified and this method gives information regarding:

○ regional wall motion;
○ myocardial thickness, mass and volume;
○ ejection fraction.

3. Volume mode

This is similar to dynamic scanning with conventional CT scanning. Following a rapid injection of contrast, continuous cross-sections are made. This allows the construction of anatomical information and is especially useful for the aorta and pulmonary arteries.

Magnetic resonance imaging

Many cardiac MRI techniques are available depending upon the way the MRI information has been derived and processed. By use of ECG-gating of the radiofrequency pulses, sequential images can be produced.

Some of the sequences which are of use in adults with congenital heart disease include:

1. Spin-echo sequencing

In images obtained by this method, moving blood gives no signal (appears as a black void) and tissues give signals which vary in shade from grey to white. This gives information regarding:

○ anatomy (see Figure 1);
○ global and regional wall motion;
○ stroke volume and ejection fraction.

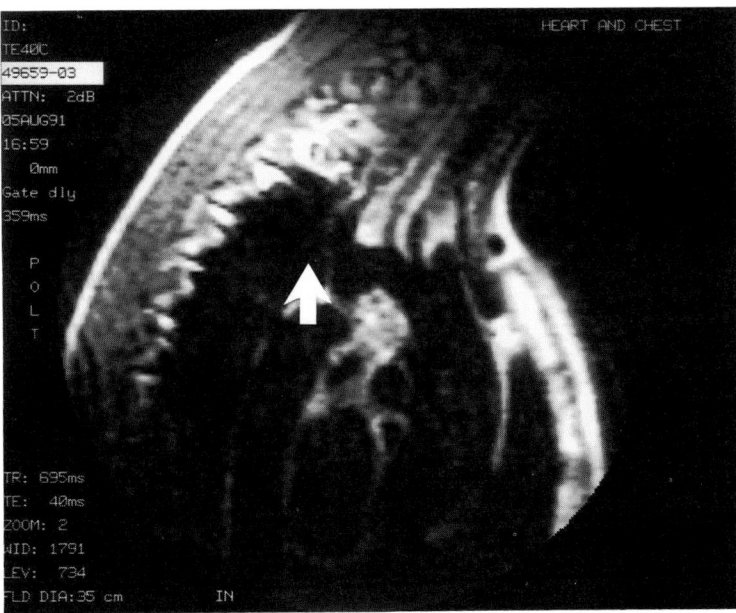

Figure 1. MRI scan from a 32-year-old with near atresia of the aortic arch at the site of discrete coarctation.

2.   Gradient-echo sequencing (also termed Cine MRI or Cine-flow MRI).

In these sequences, moving blood is associated with a high signal (appears white). Rapid sequences of images are obtained, and by modification of gradient echo, a technique known as **velocity mapping** is derived. The images show blood velocity and can be used to obtain qualitative and quantitative information regarding:

○   valvular function (e.g. stenosis or regurgitation);
○   blood flow, including intracardiac and extracardiac shunts;
○   ventricular wall motion.

3.   MRI angiography

Since flowing blood has MRI characteristics that differ from stationary tissues, it is possible to produce MRI images of flowing blood as white signals on a black background. This is mainly a research tool at present.

Patient selection, preparation and methods

For both MRI and ultrafast CT, the entire study usually takes 60–90 minutes. Patient positioning is very important in both techniques. The patient needs to be able to lie still and flat; this can be a problem, in particular with those with orthopnoea. Furthermore, the patient may be asked to hold a breath for up to 20 seconds. Some patients find the scanner claustrophobic (see below), and the MRI scanner in particular is noisy in operation. Sedation is rarely necessary, however. In CT, the patient is given a bolus of iodinated contrast into a peripheral vein. The dose of contrast used is usually 0.3–0.5 ml/kg, but up to 1 ml/kg is needed in patients with large shunts. No contrast agent is needed in MRI because of the natural contrast between flowing blood and tissues.

Advantages and disadvantages of MRI and CT

Since echo Doppler can provide excellent high quality assessment of congenital heart disease from the fetus to the adult, the use of MRI and CT must be to some extent individualized. There are particular strengths and weaknesses of the two techniques however.

Advantages

1. The techniques are non-invasive and safe. They have low morbidity and risks. No ionizing radiation or contrast is used in MRI and it has no known risks.
2. Excellent 3D images are obtained in many planes (many not available with echo Doppler). This allows the reconstruction of complex anatomy.
3. The techniques are independent of, and unlimited by, the quality of the acoustic windows, unlike echo Doppler.
4. Patients with distorted postoperative anatomy can be evaluated.
5. Information can be derived in regions which are difficult to image with echo Doppler in the adult, e.g. the aortic arch and descending aorta.
6. There is no problem with overlap of anatomical structures.
7. A single study can give a wide breadth of information regarding anatomy, blood flow, shunts, cardiac motion, etc.
8. Information can be obtained regarding the thorax and abdomen (e.g. visceral situs and postoperative pathology).

Limitations

1. Claustrophobia and patient anxiety. This is reported in approximately 5% of patients undergoing MRI and 1–2% can't complete the study. The problem is reduced by careful patient preparation and explanation, shorter scan times and the use of mirrors and microphones to allow the patient to communicate with the operator while in the scanner. In adults, sedation is usually not needed; general anaesthetic very rarely.
2. The techniques are difficult to use in very sick patients and in the immediate postoperative period.
3. Expense. The technologies are costly and still limited to a few specialized centres.
4. Patient positioning and cooperation. Some patients find it very difficult to lie flat for up to 90 minutes and hold their breath for up to 20 seconds.
5. Image artefacts, due to implanted metal prostheses, patient movement as in breathing, or to cardiac motion (reduced by ECG-gating).
6. Frequent arrhythmias can interfere with ECG-gating.
7. Relatively high doses of X-rays and contrast in ultrafast CT.
8. Contraindicated in special patient situations, where echo Doppler can be used, e.g. pregnancy and cardiac pacemakers (see below).
9. The coronary arteries are poorly visualized. Currently, the best MRI single breath-hold techniques will visualize the first one-third of the course of the epicardial coronary arteries.
10. MRI is not good in the fossa ovalis or membranous ventricular septum regions, as low signal intensity is obtained from these thin structures. As with echo Doppler, it can be hard to differentiate the normal thin fossa ovalis from a small secundum atrial septum defect (ASD).

11. Cardiac valves. MRI is not good at showing anatomical detail but can give quantitative data regarding pressure gradients across stenotic valves, and can show regurgitant valves. The opposite is true of ultrafast CT.

Special patient factors and safety considerations

There are certain specific situations where MRI and CT should be avoided or used with particular care. The special considerations for the use of ultrafast CT relate mainly to the use of relatively high doses of X-rays and the need for intravenous contrast. For MRI, the considerations relate primarily to the effects of the magnetic fields used upon ferromagnetic and electronic devices which the patient may have had implanted.

Patients with metal implants

The MRI magnets attract ferromagnetic objects, and so caution should be employed in the presence of iron-containing or other ferromagnetic objects. This is especially true in patients with implanted metallic objects which could undergo undesirable distortion or movement in a strong magnetic field. Metal objects are not a contraindication to ultrafast CT, although, as with MRI studies, they may produce some image artefact. Certain specific situations are discussed below.

Surgical clips and sutures: chest, abdomen, head

Sternotomy wires and surgical clips in the chest or abdomen are usually made of surgical stainless steel and are often only weakly ferromagnetic. These often also become rapidly immobilized postoperatively by the development of surrounding fibrous tissue. Patients with these implants can be studied by MRI without danger.

Intracranial aneurysm clips do not become immobilized by fibrous tissue, and are a contraindication to scanning. Non-ferromagnetic clips are now available, but scanning should be avoided unless it is certain that these have been used.

Prosthetic heart valves

Modern prosthetic valves contain little ferromagnetic material as stainless steel is used and this can be scanned safely. Older valves manufactured before 1964 (e.g. the old Starr-Edwards valves, pre-6000 model) do contain substantial ferromagnetic material, and patients with these should only be MRI scanned if the valve type has been previously evaluated and shown to exhibit acceptable torquing in the magnetic field of the desired strength.

Cardiac pacemakers

These are contraindications to MRI. This is related not so much to movement effects of the pacemaker (which is usually held stable in place by fibrotic tissue) but to the possibility that the electronic programming of the pacemaker can be affected by the magnetic signals. This may theoretically result in:

1. Permanent damage to the pacemaker's electronic circuits.
2. Activation of the reed switch of the pacemaker, causing it to pace in the asynchronous mode.
3. Induction of currents in the pacemaker lead, due to the magnetic field gradients, could be incorrectly sensed as cardiac activity, inhibiting the pacemaker.
4. Induction of currents in the pacing wires by the magnetic field gradients which could cause electrical stimulation of the heart.

It should be noted that we have studied many patients who have had temporary wires left under the skin after surgery with no ill effects.

Patients with pacemakers may safely undergo ultrafast CT.

Contrast material

Intravenous contrast is an important part of ultrafast CT, since it distinguishes flowing blood from other structures such as vessel walls, myocardium, thrombus, and mediastinal structures such as the thymus (this is particularly important in children). Contrast reactions can occur, which may be minor or major. Minor problems are frequent. Nausea and vomiting, flushing, transient hypotension and urticaria may occur. In those where a minor contrast reaction has been reported previously, a low-osmolar non-ionic contrast should be used (e.g. Omnipaque) and the patient should be pretreated with intravenous hydrocortisone 100 mg and chlorpheniramine 10 mg.

Major anaphylactic reactions which may be fatal are thankfully rare (less than 1 in 40,000 procedures). In those with a previous severe contrast reaction, e.g. anaphylactic shock, angiooedema, bronchospasm, contrast agents are contra-indicated and MRI scanning would be a better alternative.

Pregnancy

Ultrafast CT should not be undertaken due to the relatively high doses of X-rays and the need to use contrast media.

MRI cannot be advised during pregnancy, although patients have undergone scanning during all three trimesters without obvious ill-effects upon the mother, fetus or infant. When maternal well-being requires diagnostic studies, MRI is preferable to methods that require X-rays, such as CT or angiography.

Specific indications for MRI and CT in congenital heart diseases in the adult

In general, abnormalities of the atria, atrial septum atrioventricular valves and ventricular septum will be better demonstrated by transoesophageal echo when transthoracic imaging is inadequate. There are some specific indications for MRI and CT, however.

Great vessels

Diseases of the aorta are where these techniques, particularly MRI, really come into their own. While echo is useful for studying abnormalities of the ascending aorta, it often provides poor visualization of the aortic arch and descending aorta, particularly after surgery. Both MRI and ultrafast CT can provide excellent anatomical information regarding the aorta because of its relative immobility, the independence of acoustic windows and overlying structures of MRI and CT and the contrast between the vessel wall and flowing blood.

Aortic abnormalities which additional information can be expected from MRI and CT include:

○ coarctation of the aorta, pre- and postoperative,
○ aortic dissection
○ aortic abscess
○ aortic aneurysms
○ Marfan's syndrome

MRI is particularly valuable in patients with coarctations, preoperatively and after interventions such as balloon dilatation or surgical repair. It provides precise anatomical information and can also estimate the pressure gradient across any stenosis.

MRI detects aortic dissections with a high degree of accuracy and can show the involvement of other vessels. The entry and exit points are more difficult but associated aortic regurgitation is well shown and quantified. The involvement of the coronary arteries is not well shown. MRI is at least as sensitive as ultrafast CT but no contrast is needed. It can, however, be hard to get a sick patient into the scanner. MRI compares well with transoesophageal echo Doppler in the detection of aortic dissection, with similar sensitivity but higher specificity and with better detection of thrombus. The ability to measure velocities in the two lumens with MRI provides additional information, such as whether the false lumen is needed to supply vital organs.

MRI is ideal for the long-term follow-up of patients with Marfan's syndrome. Cine MRI and MRI angiography, in particular, allow serial non-invasive assessment of aortic root size, the presence and degree of aortic regurgitation and mitral regurgitation, left ventricular size and function, and aortic dissection, to which these patients are particularly prone.

Ultrafast CT and MRI are also useful in defining proximal pulmonary arterial anatomy, for example in patients with pulmonary atresia. The techniques are of particular value in the planning stages of surgery and in those with poor acoustic windows where echo Doppler does not provide good anatomical information. However, most of these patients will ultimately require angiography.

Pre- and postoperative assessment of complex cardiac lesions

This is another important use for these techniques. In the rare unoperated adult with tetralogy of Fallot, for example, ultrafast CT and MRI can be used to assess the size and location of the ventricular septal defect, the anatomy of the main, right and left pulmonary arteries, their size and patency, the degree of right ventricular outflow tract obstruction and, from MRI, an estimate of the severity of pulmonary stenosis can be made. Pulmonary regurgitation can be measured using MRI flow sequences, but this remains investigational at present.

In older patients, the quality of the images obtained is often superior to echocardiography. With improving MRI techniques, it may become possible to show coronary anatomy, for example, to detect the small proportion of patients where the left anterior descending coronary artery arises from the right coronary artery and crosses the right ventricular outflow tract.

Like echocardiography, MRI can show postoperative chamber size and shape, but is less good than the former at showing valvular anatomy and function. MRI is especially good postoperatively where intra- or extracardiac shunts have been produced by the construction of conduits or baffles in an effort to redirect blood flow into a more physiological manner although anatomy remains distorted. Examples are in the postoperative assessment of patients following the Fontan procedure (connection of right atrium to pulmonary artery in, e.g. tricuspid atresia), Rastelli (conduits to redirect blood at ventricular and great arteries level in patients with transposition of the great arteries with ventricular septal defect and pulmonary stenosis), Mustard or Senning (atrial baffle redirecting venous inflow within the atria in transposition) or in aorticopulmonary shunts such as Blalock, Waterston, Potts and Glenn. MRI allows careful serial follow-up of these baffles and conduits, and has made 'diagnostic' cardiac catheterization a thing of the past.

Venous return

Systemic and pulmonary venous drainage can be demonstrated by ultrafast CT, especially with subtraction techniques.

MRI can show azygos continuation of the inferior vena cava, which can be hard to detect by echocardiography in older patients. Because the inferior vena cava does not enter the heart directly, femoral cardiac catheterization can be difficult. It should also be possible to demonstrate persistence of a left-sided superior vena cava. This is particularly important as it can cause problems with cardiopulmonary bypass or can connect directly into the left atrium with consequent shunting.

MRI is not usually needed for the primary diagnosis of total anomalous pulmonary venous drainage, as this most often presents in childhood and can be diagnosed by echo Doppler. However, MRI is useful in the follow-up of older patients after corrective surgery, and in the primary diagnosis and follow-up of adults with partial anomalous pulmonary venous drainage.

Physiology of blood flow, pressure and cardiac function

Ultrafast CT and MRI are very promising as tools for cardiac functional assessment. They provide a virtual real-time method of assessing global and regional ventricular function which give results similar to invasive ventriculography. Qualitative evaluation can be made of overall ventricular function from systolic and diastolic images in the long-axis, short-axis and four-chamber views. Left and right ventricular ejection fractions can be calculated from sets of images using Simpson's rule, and the results compare well with other techniques. Regional wall motion can be assessed particularly well by cine MRI, using either a multislice technique or cine MRI with a breath-hold of 20 seconds. Ultrafast CT and MRI are especially well-suited for the assessment of right ventricular function, both pre- and postoperatively.

Ultrafast CT is good at determining flows such as cardiac output and pulmonary flow, in showing the sites of intracardiac shunts and in quantitating the size of the shunt. Using short scan times, a contrast bolus can be followed in and out of a region of interest. Contrast clearance curves are then generated by computer and the area under the curve measured. The cardiac output can be derived from the standard Stewart–Hamilton equation.

Shunt size and size evaluation is an important capability of ultrafast CT. With catheter studies and flow phantoms, the technique's accuracy has been validated and in the range 1.3:1 and 2.5:1, there is good correlation with invasive data from oximetry. Occasionally, ultrafast CT will show small shunts not detected by oximetry.

Because MRI is intrinsically sensitive to blood flow, it is highly suited to study disease states affecting flow. Flow measurements by MRI are accurate and allow the determination of cardiac output and the pulmonary/systemic flow ratio in shunts (Q_P/Q_S). MRI can also detect turbulence across stenotic valves, surgical conduits or coarctation, and a pressure gradient can be estimated accurately. Similarly, valvular regurgitation can be detected by MRI but it is only rarely that it is additive to information obtained by conventional Doppler studies.

Future prospects

MRI and ultrafast CT technology is advancing at a rapid rate. Promising prospects include the following:

1. Faster scanning techniques (subsecond imaging). The fastest current techniques (such as echoplanar MRI) are already virtually real-time.
2. Improved non-invasive angiography. Particular interest is focused upon the coronary arteries, and some promising results are emerging using MRI during a 20-second breath-hold.
3. Cine CT and cine MRI stress studies, for example using pharmacological stress with dobutamine.
4. Myocardial perfusion imaging, using MRI with contrast agents.
5. Studies of tissue characterization and examination of tissue biochemistry and metabolism with MRI.

Conclusion

MRI and ultrafast CT are useful adjuncts to echo Doppler and occasionally all three techniques are indicated in the same patient. While both MRI and ultrafast CT can give anatomical and functional information, MRI is probably the more powerful technique in that it allows certain additional assessments such as pressure gradients across valves or in vessels or surgical conduits.

Their major uses at present are in:

1. Patients with a poor acoustic window where echo Doppler is difficult.
2. The assessment of patients with aortic disease.
3. The follow-up of postoperative patients, especially in those with surgical baffles, conduits and/or distorted postoperative anatomy.

Key references

Eldredge WJ (1991) Comprehensive evaluation of congenital heart disease using ultrafast computed tomography. In Marcus ML, Schelbert HR, Skorton DJ, Wolf GL (eds) *Cardiac Imaging. A Companion to Braunwald's Heart Disease*. WB Saunders, Philadelphia.

Fisher MR, Higgins CB (1987) Magnetic resonance and cine computed tomography. In Roberts WC (ed.) *Adult Congenital Heart Disease*. FA Davis, Philadelphia.

Nitter-Haugue S, Allison D (eds) (1991) *Cardiac Imaging: X-ray, MR and Ultrasound*. Elsevier Science, Amsterdam.

Pannell DJ, Underwood SR (1993) Magnetic resonance imaging of the heart. *Br J Hosp Med* **49**(2): 90–102.

Smith WL, Stanford W, Skorton DJ, Wolk GL (1991) Assessment of congenital heart disease by nuclear magnetic resonance imaging. In Marcus ML, Schelbert HR, Skorton DJ, Wolf GL (eds) *Cardiac Imaging. A Companion to Braunwald's Heart Disease*. WB Saunders, Philadelphia.

Toombs BD (1990) Computed tomography. In Garson A, Bricker JT, McNamara DG (eds) *The Science and Practice of Paediatric Cardiology*. Lea and Febiger, Malvern, Pennsylvania.

Vick GW, Rokey R, Johnston DL (1990) Nuclear magnetic resonance and positron emission tomography – clinical aspects. In Garson A, Bricker JT, McNamara DG (eds) *The Science and Practice of Paediatric Cardiology*. Lea and Febiger, Malvern, Pennsylvania.

6

Diagnostic Cardiac Catheterization and Angiography

Introduction

Just as in paediatric congenital heart disease, the increasing utility of less invasive diagnostic methods has reduced the need for cardiac catheterization in adults with congenital heart disease. It is perhaps not an over-statement to suggest that cardiac catheterization should now no longer be required to establish the basic morphological diagnosis. Rather, cardiac catheterization should be directed to answering specific morphological or haemodynamic questions that arise from the less invasive studies. Too often, cardiologists with little experience of congenital heart disease will perform a cardiac catheterization in a patient with a difficult morphological problem because of difficulties of interpretation of the non-invasive tests. The end result is an immaculate coronary arteriogram, an inadequate left ventriculogram, and nonsensical haemodynamics. This should be a thing of the past. Cardiac catheterization has specific strengths and when capitalized upon will be complementary to the other techniques.

Procedural considerations

A biplane cine angiographic system with on-line digital subtraction angiography is ideal. The operator, radiographer, nurse and technician should have experience of cardiac catheterization in patients with congenital heart disease.

Most studies can be performed in the non-anaesthetized patient in the normal way. This has obvious advantages, but some disadvantages. Some of these studies are prolonged and, as a result, physically uncomfortable. The contrast dose may be large, further adding to the discomfort and, finally, specific investigations may be intolerable in the conscious patient (e.g. pulmonary venous wedge injection). It is therefore our policy to use general anaesthesia whenever an intervention is contemplated (see below), or if a procedure is likely to be prolonged, uncomfortable or complicated. A final consideration in this regard is the use of transoesophageal echocardiography. More and more frequently we perform this at the time of cardiac catheterization, on induction of anaesthesia. This is particularly useful for younger adolescent patients who do not tolerate the procedure so well with simple sedation and again leads to a more focused cardiac catheterization protocol. If performed under general anaesthesia, particular attention to the position of the patient is required. The arms should be raised above the head, but with the elbows elevated no higher than the nose, and fixed in a fully *adducted* position, to relieve any stretch on the brachial plexus.

The maintenance of adequate hydration is also important in these patients, especially in the presence of polycythemia. Intravenous fluids should be started before the procedure if necessary, and should be continued until the patient is tolerating oral fluids. Anticoagulants should be stopped 48 hours prior to the procedure so that the INR is less than 2 at the time of the study. If necessary, systemic heparinization will be required in the interim.

Haemodynamic measurements

While it is possible to obtain reasonable Doppler estimates of intracardiac and intravascular pressures and gradients, the gold standard remains the measurement made at the time of cardiac catheterization. Often the most critical measurement is the assessment of pulmonary arterial pressure and pulmonary vascular resistance. There is no substitute for a direct measurement of both right and left pulmonary arterial pressures when such a measurement is critical to the preoperative assessment of a patient (prior to the Fontan procedure for example). Most patients will have direct access to the pulmonary arteries, either directly, or indirectly through shunts. With normally related great vessels it is usually possible to enter the pulmonary artery antegradely from a transvenous approach. When the great vessels are transposed (in association with double inlet left ventricle for example) it is sometimes easier to enter the pulmonary artery using a retrograde arterial approach, looping a balloon tipped catheter in the ventricle backward to the pulmonary artery (Figure 1). Traversing surgically created shunts is rarely a problem, but it is worth remembering that small 'paediatric catheters', e.g. 4 or 5 French catheters, will traverse long and narrowed stenotic areas more easily than standard adult-sized catheters. Following measurements of the haemodynamics a more suitable angiographic catheter can be replaced over an exchange guide wire if necessary. If disconnected or if there is a significant stenosis between the two, then each pulmonary artery needs to be assessed individually. Occasionally, there will be no direct access to a pulmonary artery. Under these circumstances a reasonable assessment of the pulmonary arterial pressure can be obtained using a pulmonary venous approach. Using an end-hole catheter wedged in an appropriate pulmonary vein, the distal pulmonary arterial pressure on that side can be assessed in a similar fashion to the use of a pulmonary *arterial* capillary wedge assessment of left atrial pressure.

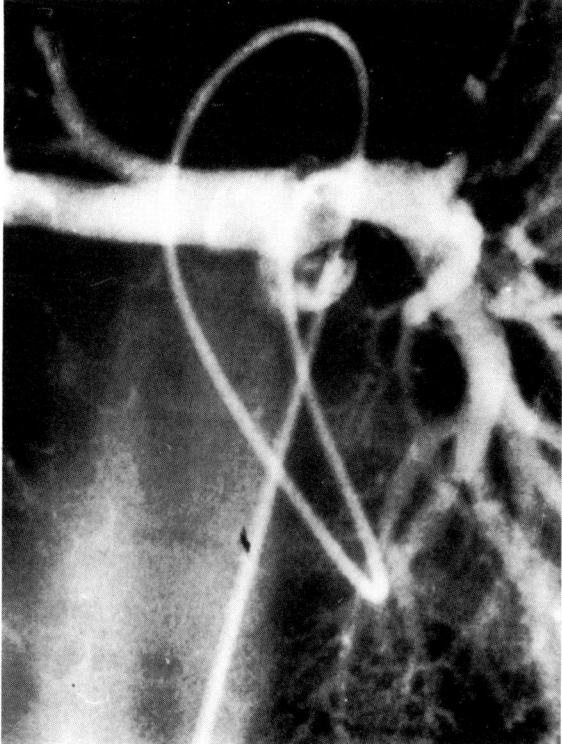

Figure 1. Pulmonary arteriogram in a patient with complex intracardiac anatomy and transposed great vessels. The easiest method of access to the pulmonary artery is demonstrated here. A retrograde arterial balloon-tipped catheter has been passed via the aorta into the right ventricle, through the ventricular septal defect and into the posteriorly placed pulmonary artery (see text for details).

It should be possible to measure all other haemodynamics in the normal way. There is a general rule: if there is a chamber measure the pressure in it, and if there is a surgical anastomosis measure the potential pressure gradient across it.

Angiography (Table 1)

There are two major errors made by inexperienced operators when dealing with adult patients with congenital heart disease. Paediatric cardiologists tend to choose a catheter size that is inadequate, and adult cardiologists choose contrast volumes that are too small. Ventriculography is now rarely required. The full sequential diagnosis should be established prior to the cardiac catheterization procedure. Sometimes, an additional ventricular septal defect will need to be excluded, or the diagnosis of the ventriculoarterial connection or relationships refined. Too often, ventriculography under these circumstances is inadequate.

Table 1. Indications for specific angiographic views

Site	Views	Dose (ml/kg)
Innominate vein	Direct AP and lateral	0.5
Superior vena cava	Direct AP and lateral	0.5
Inferior vena cava	Direct AP and lateral	0.5–1
Azygous vein	20° left or right oblique depending on position	0.5–1
Left ventricle (inlet VSD)	Straight lateral or 30° RAO Four-chamber projection	1–2
Left ventricle (outlet VSD)	30° RAO Long axis projection	1–2
Aorta (aortic regurgitation)	30° RAO Straight lateral	
Aorta (coarctation)	20° LAO Straight lateral	
Right ventricle (subpulmonary obstruction)	30° RAO Straight lateral	1
Right ventricle (valvar/supravalvar stenosis)	Four chamber Straight lateral	1
Pulmonary artery (bifurcation)	Four chamber Straight lateral	0.5
Pulmonary artery (right)	30° RAO Straight lateral	0.5–1
Pulmonary artery (left)	30° LAO Straight lateral	0.5–1
Pulmonary venous wedge	Four-chamber Straight lateral	1

There is rarely a place for performing a non-subtracted ventriculogram with less than 1 ml/kg of contrast. Thus 70–100 ml of contrast may be needed for a single injection. This can only be adequately delivered through large angiographic catheters. In the presence of a large left to right shunt, systemic ventriculography with 1–2 ml/kg of contrast may be required to demonstrate adequately the anatomy. These volumes are way in excess of those used during standard adult cardiac catheterization, but this should not deter the operator.

More usually, ventriculography is not required, but angiography will be necessary to demonstrate pulmonary arterial anatomy, systemic and pulmonary venous return, and occasionally coronary arterial anatomy in patients with complex cyanotic congenital heart disease. Systemic venous injections rarely require more than 0.5 ml/kg of contrast, and depending on the size of the pulmonary arteries 0.25–1 ml/kg of contrast per injection will be required to delineate the pulmonary arterial anatomy. Small aortopulmonary collateral arteries will be shown with smaller injections still, and sometimes these are better shown with hand injections rather than a power injection. This is particularly the case if they are stenosed or partially occluded by the passage of the catheter. Under all of these circumstances the facility for performing digital subtraction angiography is a real bonus. Smaller contrast volumes can be used, and a better demonstration of the segmental anatomy of the pulmonary vascular bed, or the exact nature of the pulmonary venous return on the laevo-phase of a pulmonary arterial injection will be obtained.

Finally, there are some specific indications for coronary arteriography. The presence of coronary arterial fistulae should be excluded when there is pulmonary atresia with intact septum (where the communication will be with the right ventricular cavity) and in any other patient with prolonged cyanosis, particularly when there is pulmonary atresia with ventricular septal defect where acquired coronary to pulmonary arterial fistulous communications may be encountered. The course of the coronary arteries may also be important. This is particularly relevant when right ventricular outflow tract surgery may be required. In 3–5% of patients with tetralogy of Fallot, for example, the distal portion of the left anterior descending coronary artery arises from the right coronary artery and traverses the right ventricular outflow tract, making placement of an outflow tract patch difficult. A particularly useful view under these circumstances is the

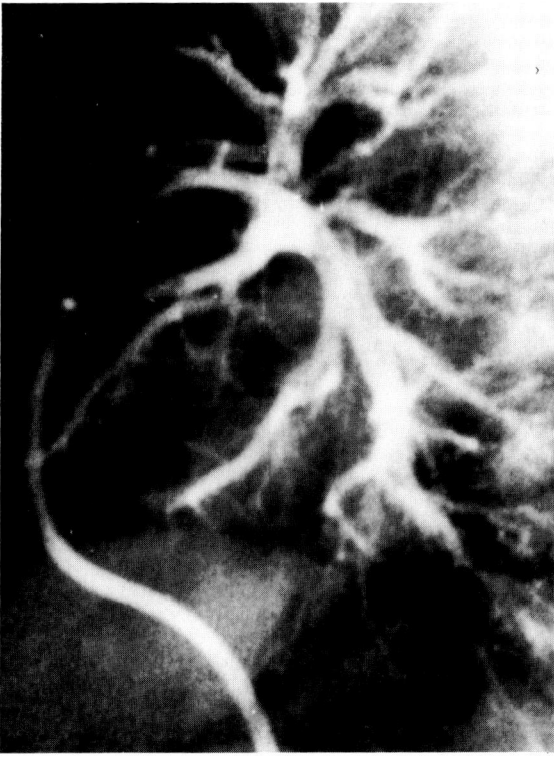

Figure 2. A pulmonary venous wedge injection. Almost all of the distribution of the left pulmonary artery is seen by a retrograde injection into the left lower pulmonary vein. The transvenous catheter has passed through the right atrium, atrial septum and is 'wedged' in the pulmonary vein (see text for details).

30° left oblique with caudocranial tilt, which will show vessels passing anterior to the right ventricular outflow tract, which ideally is itself delineated by the position of a second catheter.

Finally, if the pulmonary arteries cannot be entered directly and their demonstration is critical to the management of the patient then a pulmonary venous wedge injection will sometimes show a pulmonary artery that is not visible either echocardiographically or with magnetic resonance scanning. An angiographic catheter with an end-hole is wedged in a pulmonary vein and a relatively slow injection of 0.5–1 ml/kg of contrast given by pressure injection. This will delineate the distal pulmonary arterial anatomy and sometimes fill the pulmonary artery in its entirety, particularly if there is very sluggish flow within it (Figure 2). It is not without hazard however. An alveolar blush is uniform, and in the conscious patient (and sometimes in the anaesthetized patient) it will lead to violent coughing. Pulmonary haemorrhage with haemoptysis, and pneumothorax are also significant complications of the technique. None the less, when necessary it is a valuable additional diagnostic tool.

Conclusions

1. If in doubt, do not do it – ask an expert.
2. If in doubt, use a general anaesthetic.
3. Haemodynamics; if in doubt measure it. You never know when a particular saturation or pressure measurement may become relevant in the light of other investigations.
4. Angiography; if in doubt give more contrast rather than less. A second injection with more contrast will always cause more problems than one slightly over-compensated injection.

Section 2
Natural and Unnatural History

Cyanotic heart disease

7 Tetralogy of Fallot

Introduction

Tetralogy of Fallot is the commonest of all cyanotic congenital heart diseases, and was one of the first successfully to be 'corrected'. Although presentation beyond the first year of life is now rare, some unoperated older children and adults will be encountered. There are, however, increasing numbers of well-palliated and previously surgically corrected patients entering adult life.

Key anatomical features

The fundamental abnormality which explains most of the features of tetralogy of Fallot is that of anterior and cephalad deviation of an enlarged outlet septum. Thus, there is usually a large single perimembranous outlet ventricular septal defect with the aorta overriding the crest of the ventricular septum, and a varying degree of right ventricular outflow tract obstruction due to hypertrophy of the outlet septum and septoparietal trabeculations of the right ventricular free wall beneath a usually stenotic pulmonary valve (Figure 1). As a result, the pulmonary arteries will vary in size from diminutive, to enlarged. The right ventricular outflow tract obstruction may be progressive, and acquired pulmonary atresia (in a patient with a previously patent right ventricular outflow tract) is sometimes seen. In the unoperated state pulmonary blood supply is usually antegrade through the right ventricular outflow tract. In some patients, there will be congenital aortopulmonary collaterals leading to a multifocal pulmonary blood supply. This is much less commonly encountered than in those born with infundibular pulmonary atresia.

All patients with chronic cyanosis may develop acquired aortopulmonary collateral vessels, and patients with tetralogy of Fallot are no exception. Abnormalities of the left ventricle and left ventricular outflow tract are rare, but progressive aortic dilatation may occur with age, and a significant proportion of unoperated patients will develop some degree of aortic incompetence with time. Other rare associations with tetralogy of Fallot that are more frequently

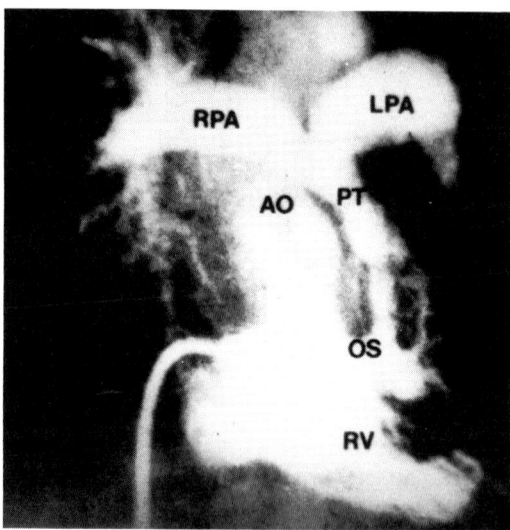

Figure 1. Right ventriculogram in four-chamber projection. There is severe infundibular pulmonary stenosis due to the deviated outlet septum (OS) and hypertrophied septoparietal trabeculations. As a result, the aorta (AO) fills through the ventricular septal defect. Although the pulmonary trunk (PT) is small the distal (RPA, LPA) pulmonary arteries are of good size and the patient is suitable for complete correction.

represented in the adult age group, because they lead to increased pulmonary blood flow in early life, are conditions such as aortopulmonary window, and anomalous origin of the left pulmonary artery from the ascending aorta. When left unoperated, these conditions will usually be complicated by pulmonary vascular disease in one or both lungs.

Natural history

The natural history of unoperated tetralogy of Fallot will depend on the degree and progression of right ventricular outflow tract obstruction. When severe these children will present in the neonatal period and require urgent palliative or corrective surgery. When less severe, progressive right ventricular outflow tract obstruction may lead to the development of hypercyanotic spells (periods of acute hypoxia which may be so severe as to cause important myocardial or cerebral ischaemia) and again will require surgical intervention in early life. In some patients, however, there is adequate pulmonary blood flow for many years. Mild to moderate hypoxaemia is tolerated remarkably well in these patients and their exercise tolerance and lifestyle may remain acceptable. Sudden death is unusual in these patients, but they of course remain susceptible to those conditions associated with a chronic right-to-left shunt. Progressive polycythaemia with

cerebral thrombosis and paradoxical embolism, cerebral abscess, bacterial endocarditis and progressive ventricular dysfunction are all rare, but well-recognized
complications of unoperated tetrology of Fallot. Chronic hypoxia and polycythaemia will be attenuated by previous palliative surgery but these procedures do little
to influence the incidence of paradoxical embolism and cerebral abscess and are
associated with their own problems of chronic ventricular volume overload and
detrimental changes in the pulmonary vascular bed. None the less, in the well-
balanced unoperated patient, and perfectly palliated adult in whom there are few
symptoms the decision to perform corrective surgery is largely a philosophical
one, based on the expected late deterioration in such patients rather than on data.

Palliative surgery

Most children will now be diagnosed and undergo corrective surgery within the
first year or two of life. This is a relatively new innovation, however, and many
adult patients will have undergone one or more palliative procedures, with
corrective surgery being performed at a much older age. A variety of palliative
procedures to increase pulmonary blood flow were evolved in the 1940s, 50s and
60s and all of these have been applied to the early management of tetralogy of
Fallot. The technical considerations, advantages and disadvantages are discussed
in full in Chapter 20. Those most frequently seen in the older age group will be
the classical Blalock-Taussig shunt (subclavian artery to pulmonary artery anastomosis), the Waterston shunt (right pulmonary artery to ascending aorta
anastomosis), and less commonly the Potts anastomosis (left pulmonary artery
to descending aorta anastomosis). These procedures were performed for a
variety of cyanotic conditions, but the Brock procedure was developed specifically for palliation of tetralogy of Fallot. By directly resecting muscle from the
right ventricular infundibulum and performing a pulmonary valvotomy, antegrade pulmonary blood flow was increased and cyanosis therefore relieved. This
procedure was performed without cardiopulmonary bypass, and while many
patients were successfully palliated, others either remained cyanosed or developed torrential pulmonary blood flow through the open ventricular septal defect
with development of pulmonary vascular disease. None the less, it was a
significant innovation in its day and, in modified form – sometimes known as
a 'first-stage correction' – it continues to be used as a palliative operation for
children with diminutive pulmonary arteries.

Corrective surgery

Complete correction of tetralogy of Fallot (closure of the ventricular septal
defect to incorporate the aorta into the left ventricle with enlargement of the

right ventricular outflow tract) has been performed for over 30 years. Many of the older patients therefore represent the outcome of some of the earliest open heart surgery performed. Although preoperative assessment, postoperative care, and intraoperative protection is now more sophisticated, the surgical techniques have changed relatively little. Adequate relief of the right ventricular outflow tract obstruction remains a prerequisite of a successful outcome. Resection of infundibular myocardium and patch enlargement of the outflow tract and pulmonary artery is therefore almost uniformly performed. In cases with severe hypoplasia of the main pulmonary artery, pulmonary valve and outflow tract, a transannular patch will be used to traverse the entire area of stenosis. In less severe cases, those with a near-normal sized pulmonary valve annulus and main pulmonary artery, the patch will be restricted to the outflow tract alone. Some degree of pulmonary incompetence is almost unavoidable after any corrective procedure, but clearly this is likely to be more severe when a transannular patch is placed. For this reason, particularly in the older patient, the surgeon may place a complete homograft in the outflow tract, or in small patients the outflow tract is reconstructed with homograft material incorporating a single cusp (a monocusp homograft) in an attempt to limit the amount of subsequent pulmonary regurgitation.

The surgical mortality of complete correction has progressively fallen. In most large centres the risk of death is less than 5%. The risk factors for early death in older patients undergoing complete correction are, in order of importance, small pulmonary arteries (a combined right and left pulmonary artery diameter at their first bifurcation of less than 1.5 times that of the aorta at the diaphragm), severe ventricular dysfunction, and multifocal pulmonary blood supply.

Clinical findings

Preoperative

In the rare preoperative adult the clinical findings will be similar to those found in children. There will be central cyanosis, finger and toe clubbing, and polycythaemia. There will usually be a palpable right ventricular impulse and a thrill in the pulmonary area. On auscultation the first heart sound is usually normal but the second heart sound will be single and there will be a loud ejection systolic murmur in the third left intercostal space. In general, the longer the systolic murmur the less severe the infundibular stenosis and vice versa. The murmur will radiate to the lung fields anteriorly and posteriorly, and if there are important congenital or acquired aortopulmonary collaterals this is where continuous murmurs will be heard. In some older patients, aortic root dilatation will lead to aortic incompetence which is clinically detectable.

Postoperative

In those palliated with an aortopulmonary connection (Blalock, Waterston, Potts) the physical signs will be similar to the preoperative patient but with a characteristic continuous murmur on the side of the chest appropriate to the previous surgery. In a patient who has previously undergone such a procedure, where no continuous murmur can be heard, there are two possibilities: the connection has closed, or it has led to pulmonary vascular disease with equalization of diastolic pressures in the aorta and pulmonary artery and hence no continuous murmur.

After complete correction the physical signs are quite different. The patient should be pink, normocythaemic, and clubbing will rapidly resolve. There may be a right ventricular impulse due to right ventricular dilatation and a faint thrill may be palpable in the third left intercostal space. On auscultation the first heart sound will be normal and the second heart sound will be single if a transannular patch has been placed, or it may be physiologically (albeit widely) split if the pulmonary valve has been preserved, or if a partial (monocusp) or complete homograft has been inserted. There is nearly always an ejection systolic murmur of varying intensity, and characteristically an early diastolic murmur due to some degree of pulmonary incompetence, again best heard in the third left intercostal space. Postoperative peripheral pulmonary artery stenosis will be associated with a systolic murmur over the lung field, but continuous murmurs should not be audible unless there is a surgical connection or congenital or acquired aorto-pulmonary collaterals.

Chest radiograph (Figure 2)

Preoperative

The typical preoperative radiograph from a patient with tetralogy of Fallot shows laevocardia with a right-sided aortic arch, a normal heart size but with an uptilted apex secondary to right ventricular hypertrophy, and pulmonary arterial bay (a concave outline to the left heart border because of the small main pulmonary artery segment) and decreased pulmonary vascular markings.

Postoperative

Figure 2 shows a typical chest radiograph from a patient after surgical correction of tetralogy of Fallot. Again there is laevocardia and a right-sided aortic arch, but after corrective surgery the heart size is enlarged (almost certainly due to right ventricular dilatation secondary to pulmonary incompetence), the right ventricular outflow tract is aneurysmal and calcified, and there are normal pulmonary vascular markings.

Electrocardiogram

Preoperative

This will usually show sinus rhythm with right axis deviation and clear-cut evidence of right ventricular hypertrophy. In those who have undergone palliative surgery, particularly those with a resulting large left-to-right shunt, there may be biventricular hypertrophy on voltage criteria.

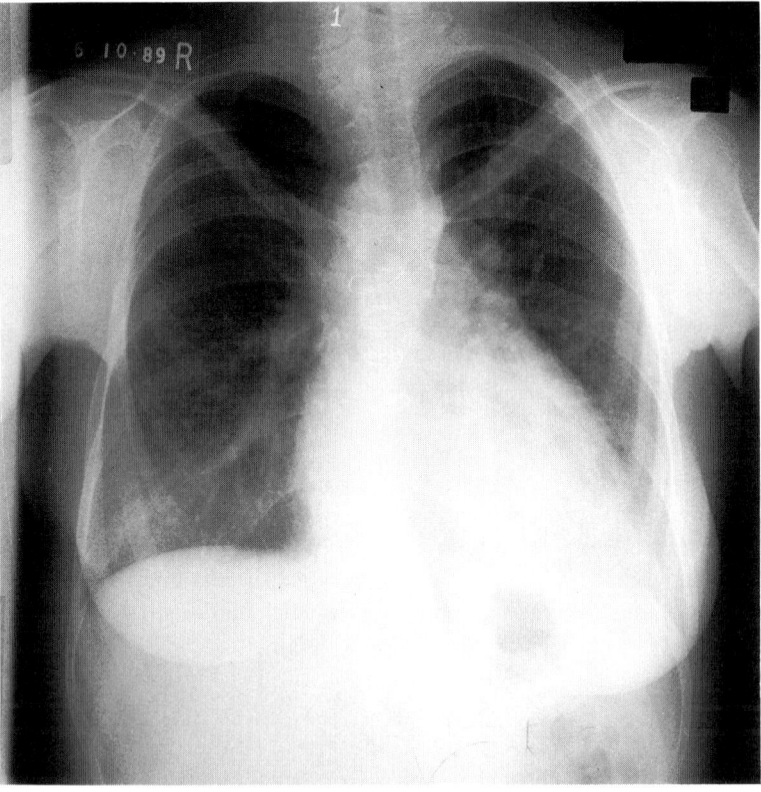

Figure 2. Characteristic chest radiograph late after repair of tetralogy. There is cardiomegaly due to right ventricular dilatation as a result of chronic pulmonary regurgitation. Note the right sided aortic arch.

Postoperative

The ECG after corrective surgery will again usually show sinus rhythm but there may be postoperative left anterior hemiblock with resulting left axis deviation. Complete right bundle branch block is the norm, although occasionally a normal QRS duration will be seen. There should be no evidence of either right or left ventricular hypertrophy unless there is a severe residual haemodynamic lesion. (Figure 3)

Cross-sectional echocardiography and Doppler studies ———

Preoperative

The preoperative echocardiographic findings are well described in conventional textbooks and will not be detailed here. However the parasternal long axis section will show a normal left ventricle, a hypertrophied right ventricle, and a single ventricular septal defect with aortic override. The parasternal short axis view should demonstrate the infundibular right ventricular outflow tract obstruction, the stenosed pulmonary valve and small main pulmonary artery. Spectral and colour Doppler will confirm a right-to-left shunt across the VSD and a large gradient across the right ventricular outflow tract. The distal pulmonary arteries are rarely well seen in adults.

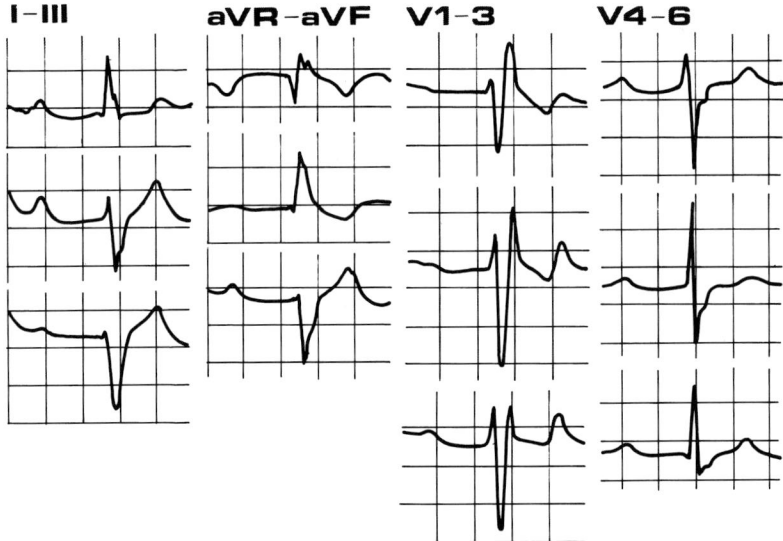

Figure 3. A postoperative electrocardiogram. There is broad complex complete right bundle branch block; left axis deviation and a prolonged PR interval. Pacing is *not* required!

Postoperative

Transthoracic echocardiography is sometimes a challenge in these older patients who have previously undergone corrective surgery. None the less, simple parasternal views will usually show the patch placed between the crest of the ventricular septum and the aortic root and in short axis the enlarged outflow tract, which may be aneurysmal. Continuous-wave Doppler will pick up even the smallest of residual ventricular septal defects, which also should be apparent clinically, and spectral and colour Doppler will demonstrate varying degrees of residual pulmonary stenosis and pulmonary regurgitation, as detailed above.

Transoesophageal echocardiography is particularly useful if a residual atrial septal defect, ventricular septal defect, or origin stenosis of one or other of the pulmonary arteries cannot be excluded using the transthoracic route.

Cardiac catheterization with angiography

Preoperative

This is required in all patients in whom corrective surgery is contemplated. Left ventriculography is required to exclude additional ventricular septal defects; aortography or selective coronary angiography is required to exclude the possibility of an anomalous coronary artery (usually the left anterior descending artery arising from the right coronary artery) traversing the right ventricular outflow tract, and in order to demonstrate the size and disposition of the pulmonary arteries. Finally, additional sources of pulmonary blood supply (acquired or congenital aortopulmonary collaterals, arterial duct) should be excluded. Haemodynamic measurements are rarely surprising. There will be evidence of a right-to-left shunt, and if it is possible to cross the right ventricular outflow tract, the pulmonary arterial pressure in unoperated patients will invariably be low. It is important to assess right and left pulmonary arterial pressures directly if palliative surgery has been performed. This is particularly important where a classical Blalock Taussig anastomosis, Waterston shunt, or Pott's anastomosis has been performed as all of these procedures may be associated with increased pulmonary blood flow and the development of pulmonary vascular disease.

Specific postoperative problems

There are two main areas of concern in the late follow-up of patients after correction of tetralogy of Fallot:

1. Arrhythmias and sudden death.
2. Right ventricular dysfunction and impaired exercise tolerance.

Arrhythmias and sudden death

Both atrial and ventricular dysrhythmias occur in these patients. Atrial flutter and fibrillation increase in frequency with the length of follow-up. Ventricular arrhythmias (Lown grade I–IV) also can be recorded with alarming frequency. To date, however, there are no prospective studies correlating abnormalities recorded on 24-hour Holter monitoring with subsequent outcome. While clearly symptomatic atrial or ventricular dysrhythmias require treatment, there is little evidence to support prophylactic drug treatment in the asymptomatic. Those at most risk of life-threatening dysrhythmias appear to be those who are operated upon later in life (over five years of age) and those with significant residual haemodynamic lesions (severe pulmonary incompetence with right ventricular dilatation, severe residual pulmonary stenosis, severe ventricular dysfunction). There is increasing evidence to suggest that residual pulmonary incompetence with right ventricular dilatation is an important cause of ventricular dysrhythmias and in turn will make them more poorly tolerated. It is not yet known whether pulmonary valve replacement in this group of patients will modify the natural history of their dysrhythmias and it certainly cannot be recommended for this reason alone.

Exercise intolerance and ventricular dysfunction

Most studies of patients after correction of tetralogy of Fallot demonstrate diminished submaximal and maximal exercise ability compared with normal. It now appears that the single most important factor associated with impaired performance is the degree of pulmonary incompetence resulting from corrective surgery. The limitation of exercise performance probably relates to right ventricular dysfunction which in turn is related to pulmonary incompetence, there being a direct relationship between the degree of pulmonary incompetence and the degree of right ventricular dilatation in postoperative patients. Indeed, there is a loose indirect relationship between the size of the heart on a routine chest radiograph (enlargement of which is usually related to right ventricular dilatation secondary to pulmonary incompetence) and exercise capacity as measured using formal, graded exercise protocols. Conceptually, these patients should be improved by pulmonary valve replacement, but as yet there are relatively few data to support this approach. Our own anecdotal experience is that dramatic improvement in clinical well-being and exercise performance can be obtained in symptomatic patients following pulmonary valve replacement and this certainly should be considered in any case where there is gross right ventricular dilatation associated with symptomatic reduction in exercise performance.

Summary

It is important to emphasize that most adult patients should lead virtually normal lives after correction of tetralogy of Fallot. Significant symptomatic deterioration should be vigorously investigated. Symptomatic arrhythmias will require treatment, but there is little evidence to support prophylactic treatment in patients with asymptomatic, atrial or ventricular dysrhythmias. Progressive cardiomegaly on the chest radiograph may be associated with impaired exercise tolerance and pulmonary valve replacement needs to be considered in these patients.

Key references

Deanfield JE (1991) Late ventricular arrhythmias occurring after repair of tetralogy of Fallot: do they matter? *Int J Cardiol* **30**: 143–50.
Murphy JG et al (1993) Long-term outcome in patients undergoing surgical repair of tetralogy of Fallot. *N Engl J Med* **329**: 593–99.

8 Transposition of the Great Arteries

Introduction

Transposition of the great arteries (TGA), with or without ventricular septal defect, now almost invariably presents in the first days or months of life with cyanosis, heart failure or both. The current trend is towards performing a definitive corrective procedure in infancy, but in the past many different approaches have been devised. Most patients encountered in adolescence and adult life will therefore have had some form of surgical intervention. Very few will have undergone anatomic correction or the arterial 'switch' procedure (see below), however. This procedure became popular, and acceptable in terms of its mortality, in the 1980s. By far the majority of older patients will have had one of the atrial redirection procedures, which have their own late complications, the recognition and treatment of which being the key to appropriate management of this group of patients.

Key anatomic features

Simple transposition

These patients have an intact ventricular septum, or occasionally a small, haemodynamically insignificant muscular VSD. Thus, the aorta arises wholly from the right ventricle and the pulmonary artery from the left ventricle (Figure 1). Right ventricular outflow tract obstruction (subaortic stenosis) is exceptional but left ventricular outflow tract obstruction (LVOTO) is much more commonly encountered. This takes many different forms. Fixed subpulmonary obstruction may be due to a fibromuscular ridge, tissue tags or fixed 'tunnel'-like narrowing of a subpulmonary infundibulum. More frequently seen is dynamic LVOTO. This results in part from the interventricular septum being pushed backwards, towards the left ventricle due to systemic pressure in the right ventricle, but there may also be systolic anterior motion of the mitral valve indistinguishable from that seen in hypertrophic obstructive cardiomyopathy. Finally, pulmonary valve

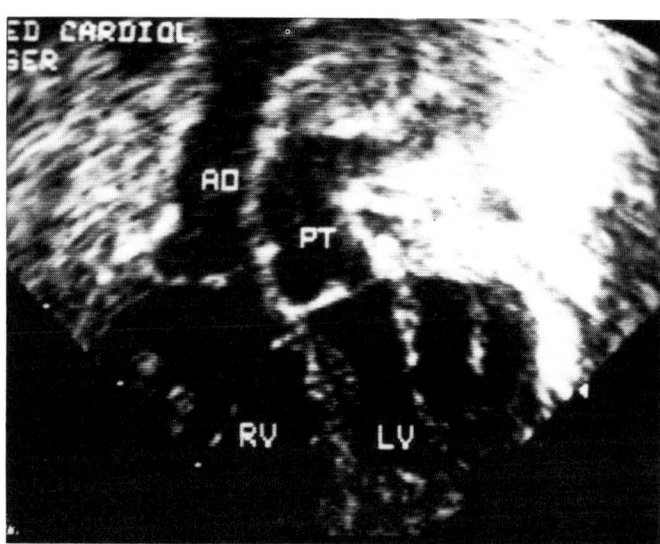

Figure 1. Cross-sectional echocardiogram showing transposition of the great arteries. The bifurcating pulmonary trunk (PT) arises from the left ventricle (LV) whereas the right sided aorta (AO) arises from the right ventricle and forms the aortic arch superiorly.

stenosis is sometimes encountered although it is rarely haemodynamically significant enough to influence early management. Survival in these patients depends on mixing of oxygenated and deoxygenated blood. Balloon atrial septostomy and prostaglandin therapy to maintain ductal patency are life-saving manoeuvres in neonates and infants, but a naturally occurring large atrial septal defect (ASD) or patent ductus arteriosus (PDA) (the latter sometimes resulting in pulmonary vascular disease) will be seen in the rarely encountered unoperated adults.

Transposition with ventricular septal defect

These patients have a haemodynamically important ventricular septal defect, either muscular or perimembranous, usually of the outlet type. Indeed, it is the disposition of the outlet septum (malalignment of which is a feature of the outlet VSD) which governs their presentation and prognosis. Again, as in simple transposition, the aorta usually arises wholly from the right ventricle. The pulmonary artery not infrequently 'overrides' the crest of the ventricular septum. The differentiation from double outlet right ventricle relies on an arbitrary 50% rule. If more than 50% of the diameter of the pulmonary artery is committed to the left ventricle then the diagnosis is TGA+VSD, whereas if more than 50% is committed to the right ventricle, then the diagnosis is double outlet right ventricle (note: this is independent of infundibular anatomy).

As mentioned earlier, it is the disposition of the outlet septum that governs the haemodynamics and prognosis in this group. It is always malaligned with respect to the rest of the ventricular septal where there is an outlet VSD. However, it may also be deviated beneath the arterial trunks. Posterior deviation beneath the pulmonary artery will restrict pulmonary blood flow and pulmonary arterial development and these patients will often present with duct-dependent pulmonary blood flow. Anterior deviation of the outlet septum will produce subaortic stenosis and hypoplasia of the aorta. Coarctation or interruption of the aorta with unimpeded pulmonary blood flow is the commonest mode of presentation in this group, and has the worst long-term prognosis.

Management of simple transposition

Early palliation

Early palliation to improve critical cyanosis requires improved mixing of systemic and pulmonary venous blood. In 1966 Rashkind introduced the percutaneous balloon atrial septostomy which transformed the early survival of patients with simple transposition (remember, this predated the introduction of prostaglandin therapy to maintain ductal patency by some 10–15 years). Prior to this a surgical septectomy was required. The Blalock Hanlon surgical septostomy is still performed in patients in whom balloon septostomy is inadequate, when the atrial septum is intact, or in patients in whom 'correction' cannot be contemplated and long-term assurance of atrial mixing is required. Arterial oxygen saturations between 60 and 80% can be expected after atrial septostomy or septectomy and this is adequate to allow virtually normal growth and normal intellectual development. A critical examination of survival after septostomy/septectomy reveals a significant attrition during the first year of life. Atrial 'corrective' surgery was traditionally performed between the ages of 6 and 12 months and the advocates of the early arterial switch emphasize the need not only to examine the surgical mortality of the atrial procedures but also the attrition prior to it being performed.

Atrial redirection procedures

A variety of approaches were developed on definitive treatment for simple transposition. Occasionally a patient will be encountered having undergone a partial repair (by design rather than mistake!). In 1956 Baffes described a baffle procedure to incorporate the right sided pulmonary veins into the pulmonary venous atrium and the IVC to the systemic venous atrium, thereby, partially relieving cyanosis. The Mustard and Senning procedures evolved from this approach, both redirecting completely the pulmonary venous return towards the systemic right ventricle by 'baffling' systemic venous blood towards the left ventricle. Although achieving a series circulation similar to normal, these procedures cannot be considered to be truly 'corrective' because the fundamental anatomic abnormality remains. Furthermore, although the surgical technique of the two major approaches differs markedly (the Mustard incorporating an artificial or pericardial intra-atrial patch, the Senning using only intra-atrial flaps) their late complications are very similar.

Post-Mustard assessment

The clinical follow-up of a patient after intra-atrial repair should be directed towards their three major complications:

○ baffle obstruction
○ arrhythmia
○ right ventricular failure

Clinical examination

Most patients will be asymptomatic. Peripheral oedema, ascites or morning eyelid oedema is strongly suggestive of severe bicaval obstruction. Obstruction or even atresia of a single limb of the baffle is rarely symptomatic as decompression via the azygous system occurs. None the less, there will usually be a raised jugular venous pressure in isolated superior caval obstruction and non-pulsatile hepatomegaly when the inferior caval channel is obstructed. Pulmonary venous obstruction is also remarkably well tolerated until severe. None the less, significant shortness of breath on exertion, orthopnoea or paroxysmal nocturnal dyspnoea should raise the possibility of either pulmonary venous obstruction or systemic ventricular failure.

Examination of the praecordium will invariably reveal right ventricular hypertrophy, with a diffusely palpable or impalpable apex beat. The aorta is anterior in the chest and so a palpable second sound is also frequently found. This also explains the very loud, and often single second heart sound on auscultation. An accentuated pulmonary component should again raise the suspicion of pulmonary venous obstruction. Just occasionally a mid diastolic murmur will be heard towards the left lower sternal border when there is severe pulmonary venous baffle obstruction but more usually there will be murmurs. More commonly, there will be murmurs of mild tricuspid regurgitation or of fixed or dynamic left ventricular outflow tract obstruction (pulmonary stenosis/subpulmonary stenosis).

Investigations

Chest radiograph

Mild to moderate cardiomegaly is the norm. A small or normal sized heart with pulmonary venous engorgement or pulmonary oedema is almost pathognomic of pulmonary venous baffle obstruction. The upper mediastinum is usually narrow (because of the anteroposterior relationship of the great arteries) but when there is superior caval obstruction the mediastinum may be widened by dilatation of the superior caval vein and azygous system.

Electrocardiogram

The resting electrocardiogram can be expected to show extreme right ventricular dominance and right axis deviation. In adults, resting sinus rhythm is the exception rather than the rule. Low atrial (as evidenced by a short PR interval and superior P wave axis) or junctional rhythm is more usual. The 24-hour Holter in these patients will usually show prompt restoration of sinus rhythm with activity. Symptomatic bradycardia is rare and syncopal episodes are more likely to be due to tachyarrhythmia. Atrial flutter (see below) is particularly poorly tolerated.

Echocardiography

These patients are often surprisingly echogenic. Subcostal imaging or a posteriorly tilted apical four chamber will best show the pulmonary venous baffle. Colour flow mapping is invaluable in assessing baffle flow. Transthoracic imaging is less satisfactory when assessing the systemic venous baffles. Again colour flow mapping may highlight areas of turbulent flow at the mouth of IVC or SVC into the systemic venous atrium. It is worth pointing out that not all turbulent flow in the systemic venous atrium is due to obstructed venous return. Even small baffle leaks, which are quite common, may give obvious high velocity Doppler signals (their flow is usually from the pulmonary venous to the systemic venous atrium) and it is easy to misinterpret this as possible obstruction. If in doubt then transoesophageal echo is the method of choice for clarifying the atrial anatomy in these patients.

Ventricular performance is very difficult to assess. Right ventricular dilatation is expected and its shortening fraction is very commonly depressed. Indeed, the appearance of the right ventricle is often one of sluggish and globally depressed function. Doppler studies frequently reveal mild tricuspid incompetence, but analysis of ventricular inflow is more difficult. Atrial systolic flow may be absent (due to junctional rhythm or atrial failure) and even when there is sinus rhythm transtricuspid and transmitral flow may be chaotic and very difficult to interpret. This is presumably owing to the influence of baffle movement and shape on the characteristics of transatrial flow. The left ventricle is usually much smaller than the right, and appears 'squashed' due to posterior displacement of the interventricular septum, which contracts with the right ventricle. Systolic anterior motion of the mitral valve will sometimes be seen under these circumstances, and large LV outflow tract gradients may be measured in the systole. A hypertrophied or dilated left ventricle is strong indirect evidence of a raised pulmonary vascular resistance, either secondary to pulmonary venous obstruction or pulmonary vascular disease.

Cardiac catheterization

There is no place for 'routine' diagnostic cardiac catheterization; a combination of transthoracic and transoesophageal echocardiography should adequately demonstrate the postoperative anatomy and physiology in most patients. However, diagnostic cardiac catheterization and angiography will be required in a few, and of course when transcatheter intervention is contemplated. Ideally, the haemodynamics should be similar to normal, although the systemic right ventricular end-diastolic pressure after the Mustard procedure is often higher than that of the normal systemic left ventricle. It is important to perform bilateral simultaneous wedge pressures versus right ventricular diastolic pressure whenever pulmonary venous obstruction is suspected. This is because unilateral

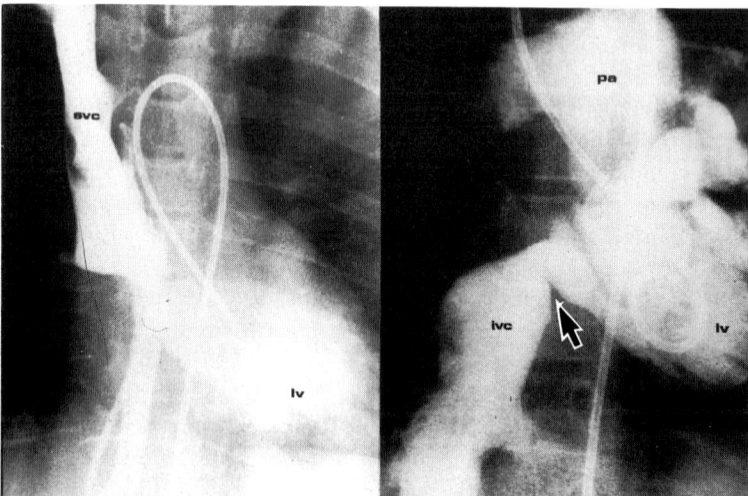

Figure 2.   Selective superior (SVC) and inferior (IVC) caval injections after the Mustard procedure. The superior channel is unobstructed, but there is a discrete narrowing of the inferior channel (arrow). lv, left ventricle; pa, pulmonary artery.

obstruction of the pulmonary veins is sometimes seen. Selective angiography in the superior and inferior caval veins should always be performed (Figure 2). As mentioned earlier, decompression of even severe obstruction of one of the limbs via the azygous system may be effective, and so there may be no measurable pressure gradient. Angiography will demonstrate the stenosis, and abnormal azygous flow under these circumstances.

Selective right and left pulmonary arterial angiography should be performed if pulmonary venous obstruction is suspected. The laevophase of these injections should demonstrate the site of obstruction but, particularly when severe, may be difficult to interpret. Interestingly, the straight lateral projection is sometimes more informative than anteroposterior or four-chamber views, but biplane angiograms should always be recorded. If any doubt remains, then a pulmonary capillary wedge pressure with simultaneous right ventricular pressure measurements should be made (Figure 3).

Interventional catheterization

Systemic venous baffle obstruction usually responds well to standard balloon dilatation although occasionally an intravascular stent will be required. Pulmonary venous obstruction is much more resistant to balloon dilatation. It is usually possible to obtain some relief by retrograde dilatation (via the tricuspid valve) using a single or two-balloon technique but it is rarely definitive and, in our hands, restenosis is almost inevitable. Direct surgical relief is usually required but it is worth considering Mustard takedown and conversion by anatomic correction

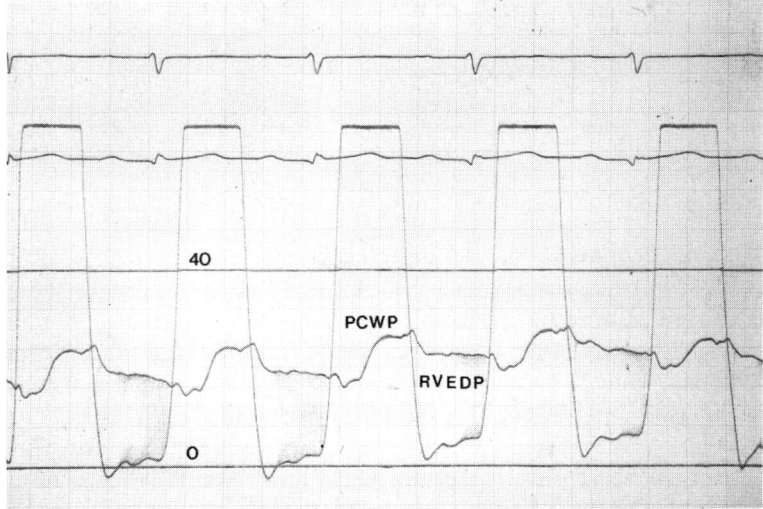

Figure 3. Simultaneous recordings of pulmonary capillary wedge and right ventricular pressures. There is a marked gradient, indicating severe pulmonary venous baffle obstruction.

(arterial switch), particularly when the left ventricular pressure has been elevated as a consequence of the severe downstream obstruction (see below).

Right ventricular failure

Concerns regarding the long-term ability of the right ventricle to support the systemic circulation were, in large part, responsible for the development of the arterial switch procedure. As mentioned above some degree of right ventricular dilation and reduction in ejection fraction is expected in these patients, but progressive deterioration (in the first one or two decades of follow-up) is really quite unusual. Exercise dysfunction is also almost uniformly reported. Maximal exercise capacity, measured formally, is reduced when compared with normal controls, but the relevance of this in the asymptomatic patient is uncertain. Again, progressive deterioration is rare and furthermore submaximal perform-ance as assessed by oxygen consumption, anaerobic threshold, etc, has been reported within normal limits in several studies. It remains to be seen whether the right ventricle will fail in a significant proportion of patients with increasing follow-up, but for the time being this remains a perhaps over-emphasized problem in these patients. None the less a small number of patients will present with significant right ventricular dysfunction (often as a consequence of pro-gressive tricuspid regurgitation). Cardiac transplantation is one option, but the possibility of Mustard takedown and arterial switch should be considered. This is particularly attractive if the left ventricle is already 'primed' to tolerate conversion to the systemic ventricle (because of severe pulmonary venous pathway obstruc-tion or dynamic LVOTO for example). Otherwise the left ventricle must be 'trained' by prior pulmonary arterial banding. This approach remains experi-mental and should be restricted to special centres, but early results are promising.

Arrhythmias

Loss of sinus rhythm on the resting electrocardiogram is frequently seen in patients after intraatrial repair. This is rarely symptomatic, indeed conversion to sinus rhythm on exercise is usually prompt. This loss of sinus node function is almost certainly due to direct surgical trauma to its blood supply and possibly the atrial conduction tracts. None the less symptomatic bradycardia is rare and only occasionally will a pacemaker be required. Tachyarrhythmias are much more sinister. Atrial flutter seems to be particularly poorly tolerated and when detected, should be vigorously treated. Atrial fibrillation is less common as are ventricular arrhythmias. None the less sudden late death does occur and a yearly 24-hour ECG recording should be part of the 'routine' assessment of even asymptomatic patients.

Transposition with ventricular septal defect ————————

Unobstructed pulmonary blood flow

This group can be further divided into those with coexistent subaortic stenosis (due to anterior deviation of the outlet septum) and those with unobstructed aortic flow. In the former, presentation is usually in the neonatal period with aortic arch obstruction. This is the group with the worst prognosis and survival into adult life following neonatal arch reconstruction is relatively rare. More commonly, there is unobstructed systemic and pulmonary arterial flow. These patients do well initially but gradually develop heart failure as the pulmonary resistance falls. Unoperated adult survivors often deny a history of early heart failure and it may be that the pulmonary vascular resistance has never fallen normally in these patients. Indeed, an occasional patient with simple transposition will develop progressive pulmonary vascular disease, in the absence of a right-to-left shunt, and there is no doubt that the pulmonary vascular bed is unusually reactive in this group of patients. For this reason patients with transposition and large VSD require surgery in infancy. Pulmonary artery banding was sometimes performed as palliation prior to a later Mustard procedure, or more often a Mustard procedure with VSD closure was performed as a primary procedure. The mortality of this procedure was high (15–25%) however, and today's approach of a primary anatomic correction with concomitant closure of the VSD has improved the outcome in this group. Survivors of the Mustard procedure have the same problems as when it is performed for simple transposition (see above). There are few data, but anecdotally these patients seem more likely to be functionally impaired and more compromised by tachyarrhythmias.

Transposition, ventricular septal defect and subpulmonary stenosis or atresia ————————

These patients represent a distinct subgroup and presentation, surgical management and outcome is quite different from that discussed above. The combination of transposition haemodynamics and reduced pulmonary blood flow usually leads to severe neonatal cyanosis. Adult survivors will almost always have undergone palliative or corrective surgery, although occasionally the systemic to pulmonary blood flow is 'balanced', particularly if there is an additional PDA for example, and unoperated survival is possible.

Palliative surgery

The whole spectrum of palliative procedures to increase pulmonary blood flow have been applied to this group (see Chapter 20). Unless complicated by the adverse effects of such palliation pulmonary artery growth is rarely limited and most ultimately become suitable for biventricular corrective surgery.

Corrective surgery

The VSD in these patients is usually large and the subpulmonary stenosis severe. The most successful and most frequently performed corrective procedure was developed by Rastelli in the late 1960s. The term 'Rastelli Procedure' is now rather loosely applied to any operation involving closure of a VSD to incorporate the aorta to the left ventricle with concomitant right ventricular-to-pulmonary artery conduit (in pulmonary atresia with VSD for instance), but it was originally described in this group of patients.

Follow-up of the Rastelli procedure

This operation is rarely performed in the first five years of life. This is because an external right ventricle-to-pulmonary arterial conduit is required. Although technically possible, early surgery will inevitably lead to acquired 'stenosis' of the conduit due to rapid somatic growth. Later surgery allows insertion of an 'adult-sized' conduit and so, in theory at least, avoids the need for conduit replacement. None the less, conduit stenosis is the single most frequently encountered late complication in these patients. This takes many forms. Anastomatic line stenosis, kinking, calcification and intimal peel are all described and vary in frequency depending on the type of conduit used.

Clinical examination

A right ventricular impulse and palpable systolic and sometimes diastolic thrill at the upper left sternal border may be present. A split second heart sound with an easily audible pulmonary component usually goes along with an unobstructed conduit, a single second sound usually implying stenosis of the connection or valve leaflet fibrosis/calcification. Exceptional patients will have no murmur, but most will have a systolic ejection murmur and early diastolic murmur reflecting some degree of stenosis and regurgitation.

Electrocardiogram

This usually shows sinus rhythm with right axis deviation. Complete right bundle branch block is usual and so makes assessment of right ventricular hypertrophy difficult.

Chest radiograph

Mild-to-moderate cardiomegaly is not unusual. Conduit calcification is frequently seen and does not necessarily imply stenosis. Unequal pulmonary vascular markings may, however, indicate branch pulmonary stenosis.

Echocardiography

The VSD patch will be seen arising from the right side of the interventricular septum and passing up to the aortic root. Because of the large size of the VSD there is rarely any left ventricular outflow tract obstruction. The main pulmonary artery is usually tied to prevent antegrade flow from the left ventricle. The high parasternal short axis view usually best shows the RV to PA connection, and provides the ideal position for Doppler interrogation of the conduit and origin of the branch pulmonary arteries. If the conduit is not well seen it is usually possible to assess the RV pressure from the tricuspid regurgitant jet that is usually present. Transoesophageal echocardiography is indicated when transthoracic imaging is suboptimal but it is sometimes difficult also to image the conduit without biplane or multiplane imaging.

Cardiac catheterization

If there is doubt about the presence of a residual ventricular septal defect, conduit stenosis, or branch pulmonary artery stenosis, then cardiac catheterization will be necessary. It is a generalization but balloon dilatation of conduit stenosis is rarely successful, and severe obstruction (systemic or suprasystemic right ventricular pressure) will usually require surgical replacement. Branch pulmonary artery stenosis is more amenable to balloon dilatation, particularly if high-pressure balloons are used. Expandable but undilatable stenoses will usually be relieved by the placement of an endovascular stent, and so avoid the need for surgery.

Key references

Kavlitz R, Stumper OF, Geuskens R et al (1990) Comparative value of the praecordial and transoesophageal approaches in the echocardiographic evaluation of atrial baffle function after an atrial correction procedure. *J Am Coll Cardiol* **16**: 686–94.

Lock JE, Bass JL, Casteneda-Zuniga W et al (1984) Dilatation angioplasty of congenital or operative narrowings of venous channels. *Circulation* **70**: 457–64.

Mahoney L, Turley K, Ebert P, Heymann M (1982) Long-term results after atrial repair of transposition of the great arteries in early infancy. *Circulation* **66**: 253–58.

Stark J, Silove ED, Taylor JFN, Graham GR, Kirklin JW (1974) Obstruction to systemic venous return following the Mustard operation for transposition of the great arteries. *J Thorac Cardiovasc Surg* **68**: 742–49.

9

Pulmonary Atresia

In collaboration with Dr S Cullen

Introduction

In congenital heart defects associated with pulmonary atresia no blood enters the pulmonary artery directly from the right ventricle. In other words there is complete obstruction to the right ventricular outflow tract. This may occur in the setting of an intact ventricular septum or in association with a ventricular septal defect. These two conditions are distinct morphological entities which require different treatment and management protocols. Pulmonary atresia with an intact ventricular septum is associated with varying degrees of hypoplasia of the right ventricle and the presence of congenital communications between the ventricular cavity and the coronary arteries (fistulae or sinusoids). The pulmonary circulation is supplied by the duct and aortopulmonary collateral arteries are very rarely seen. The degree of hypoplasia of the right ventricle and presence of right ventricular to coronary artery communications dictates the management.

In pulmonary atresia and ventricular septal defect, the pulmonary circulation may be supplied by a duct, bronchiolar collaterals, and in 60%, multiple aorto-pulmonary collateral arteries (MAPCAS) arising from the descending aorta. In this condition it is the means by which the pulmonary circulation is supplied that dictates the management.

Patients with pulmonary atresia and intact ventricular septum presenting in the neonatal period will not survive to adulthood unless surgical intervention is undertaken. However, patients with pulmonary atresia, ventricular septal defect and major aortopulmonary collateral arteries may occasionally be encountered in adult practice without having undergone previous surgery.

Key anatomical features

In pulmonary atresia and ventricular septal defect, the ventricular septal defect is of similar morphology as that encountered in tetralogy of Fallot, i.e. a large perimembranous outlet ventricular septal defect with aortic override. The pulmonary atresia is usually congenital but may be acquired. The atresia usually occurs at infundibular level or occasionally may be at the right ventricular–pulmonary trunk junction with a patent hypertrophied infundibular area. This condition is associated with major abnormalities of the pulmonary arterial tree. In the majority (70–80%) the right or left pulmonary arteries are small but confluent while in about 20–30% of cases they are non-confluent or absent. The pulmonary arteries themselves may be extremely small with abnormal branching patterns. Approximately 60% of patients have large aortopulmonary collateral arteries, supplying all or part of the pulmonary vascular bed. These occur with much greater frequency in those patients with non-confluent pulmonary arteries (~80%) as against 30–40% in those with confluent arteries, and are extremely unusual in patients with classical tetralogy of Fallot. They usually arise from the upper or mid descending thoracic aorta. Beyond their origins these collateral arteries resemble muscular systemic arteries. Multiple stenoses may occur as a result of intimal proliferation which occurs in approximately 60% of collateral arteries. The development of pulmonary vascular disease in early childhood is directly related to the number of collateral arteries and the degree of stenosis in them. In those without stenoses there is pulmonary hyperperfusion and hypertension with early progression to pulmonary vascular disease. In addition to these large aortopulmonary collateral arteries others may arise from the right or left subclavian artery usually from the side opposite the aortic arch. Finally, additional flow may occur from enlarged intercostal, bronchiolar, and internal mammary arteries.

Pulmonary atresia with intact ventricular septum is characterized by variable degrees of right ventricular and tricuspid valve hypoplasia. In the majority of patients the right ventricular cavity size is reduced, usually secondary to massive wall hypertrophy. Occasionally, in the presence of Ebstein's malformation or severe tricuspid incompetence the right ventricle may be enlarged. The wall of the right ventricle is usually heavily fibrosed. The pulmonary valve is atretic and this atresia may extend to involve the infundibular area. The pulmonary arterial trunk and pulmonary arteries are usually of near normal size. Coronary sinusoids are present in one half of patients with pulmonary atresia and intact ventricular septum and these fistulous connections may occur between the right ventricular cavity and branches of the left or right coronary artery. The smaller the right ventricular cavity, the higher the prevalence of right ventricular-to-coronary artery fistulae. In a minority of patients the coronary circulation may be derived entirely from the right ventricle (right-ventricular-dependent coronary circulations). This is particularly common when there are stenoses in the coronary arterial system and survival to adulthood is rare. In most cases the tricuspid valve is small, the right atrium is enlarged, and there must be an interatrial communication.

Natural history

In some patients with pulmonary atresia and ventricular septal defect, confluent pulmonary arteries and absence of major aortopulmonary collateral arteries, the natural history resembles that of classical tetralogy of Fallot (see Chapter 7). Complete repair with a conduit from right ventricle to pulmonary artery can be performed in most. Of the remainder, most patients present in infancy but those with large major aortopulmonary collateral arteries may escape detection until later in childhood or, rarely, adult life. Clinical presentation is dictated by the flow through major aortopulmonary collateral arteries. When there is low flow they usually present with cyanosis whereas those with larger collaterals may present with breathlessness due to increased pulmonary blood flow. With the development of stenoses of the collateral arteries, cyanosis tends to become progressive and these patients are prone to all the complications of chronic hypoxaemia and polycythaemia such as cerebral thrombosis, abcess and bacterial endocarditis. Pulmonary vascular disease may develop early in childhood in patients with a large number of major aortopulmonary collateral arteries with chronic pulmonary over-circulation. Occasionally, patients may be haemodynamically well balanced and may survive for several decades with an acceptable quality of life and exercise tolerance.

In contrast all patients with pulmonary atresia and intact ventricular septum present in the neonatal period with cyanosis. Ductal patency is essential for survival. In the absence of surgical intervention this condition is lethal in infancy. In patients with marked hypoplasia of the right ventricle and right ventricular dependent coronary artery circulation surgical intervention may not be possible and cardiac transplantation may be the only hope. No matter what the intervention, survival with a biventricular repair is possible in the minority (10–20%).

Clinical findings and investigations

In patients with pulmonary atresia and ventricular septal defect with few major aortopulmonary collateral arteries the clinical picture is dominated by cyanosis. If many collateral arteries are present, breathlessness and dyspnoea predominate, and these may be associated with failure to thrive. Continuous murmurs are heard over both lung fields. The second heart sound is single.

In pulmonary atresia and intact ventricular septum severe cyanosis develops as the duct gets smaller. The second heart sound is single and the murmur is continuous when the duct is patent.

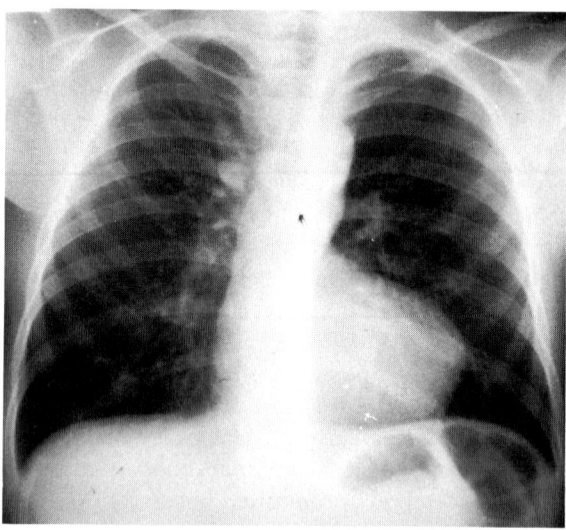

Figure 1.   Chest radiograph from a patient with pulmonary atresia, VSD and collaterals. There is an uptilted apex pulmonary artery bay and unequal pulmonary vascular markings, increased on the right.

Chest radiograph

Chest X-ray in patients with pulmonary atresia and ventricular septal defect is similar to that of patients with tetralogy of Fallot with a boot-shaped heart and absence of the pulmonary artery bay. The amount of pulmonary vascular markings is directly related to the number of MAPCAS (Figure 1). If there are few there will be pulmonary oligaemia whereas if many are present there may be multiple ill-defined parenchymal shadowing in both lung fields. The aortic arch may be right (30%) or left sided.

In patients with pulmonary atresia and intact ventricular septum heart size is usually normal or small and there is always pulmonary oligaemia.

Electrocardiogram

The electrocardiogram in pulmonary atresia and ventricular septal defect is similar to that in tetralogy of Fallot with right axis deviation and right ventricular hypertrophy. Patients with pulmonary atresia and intact ventricular septum usually have right axis deviation and left ventricular dominance.

Cross-sectional echocardiography

The diagnosis of either pulmonary atresia with ventricular septal defect or with an intact ventricular septum is readily made on cross-sectional echocardiographic examination. In the former, the presence of additional ventricular septal defects and the presence or absence of confluent pulmonary arteries should be noted. Colour Doppler examination will readily alert one to the presence of MAPCAS. In patients with pulmonary atresia and intact ventricular septum the size of the tricuspid valve and right ventricular cavity should be noted. Colour Doppler examination may show turbulent flow within the right ventricular myocardium suggesting right ventricular fistulae to the coronary arteries.

Angiography

Angiography is essential to the planning of surgical strategies for the management of patients with pulmonary atresia. In pulmonary atresia with ventricular septal defect, additional ventricular septal defects need to be excluded and the central pulmonary arteries can be evaluated for overall size, the presence of stenoses, and non confluence. The main purpose in most patients, however, is to precisely define the multifocal blood supply to the lungs (Figure 2). The circulation to each lobe and segment of the lung must be defined angiographically in order to plan repair. Injection of contrast material into each of the individual collaterals is required. Because of the complexity of the anatomy in some patients, it may not be possible to obtain all this information at a single cardiac catheterization. Occasionally, pulmonary wedge injection is necessary to define the pulmonary arteries (see Chapter 6), usually noted by their seagull appearance and separation from the main cardiac silhouette. If a multifocal source of blood supply to individual lobes is detected it may be possible to

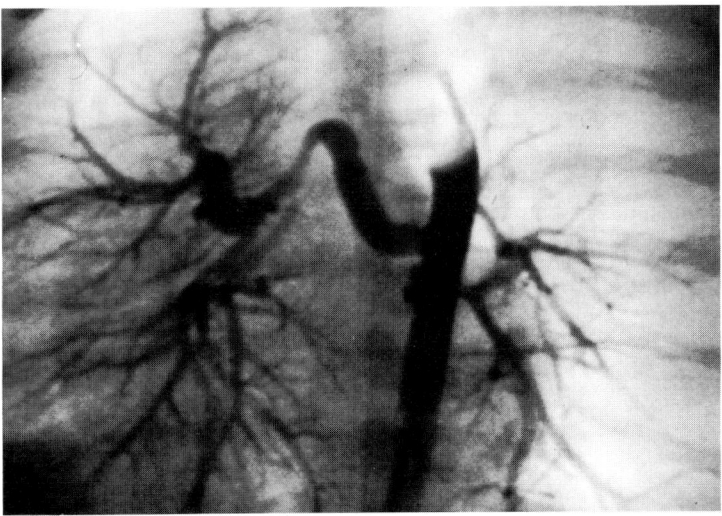

Figure 2. Balloon occlusion aortogram showing multiple aortopulmonary collateral arteries. Note the stenosis in the large collateral supplying most of the right lung.

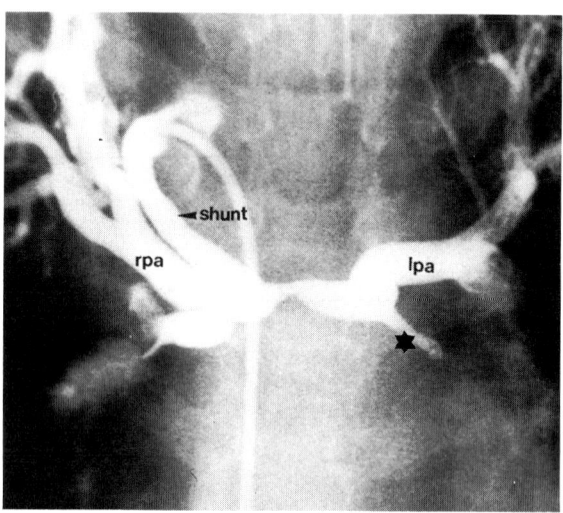

Figure 3.   The central pulmonary arteries in a patient with pulmonary atresia, ventricular septal defect and multiple aortopulmonary collaterals. There is an injection into a modified Blalock Taussig shunt. The central pulmonary arteries fill (as does the diminutive main pulmonary artery *), but note that there is no direct supply to either lower lobe.

occlude the collateral vessels with coils at the time of cardiac catheterization (Chapter 19). This is only possible if there are pulmonary arterial vessels supplying the same area as the collateral and balloon occlusion does not result in a dangerous fall in oxygen saturation. In addition to the delineation of the collateral arteries, the presence of peripheral pulmonary stenoses and indeed stenoses in the collateral arteries themselves should be documented (Figure 3). These may be amenable to balloon dilatation or transcatheter placement of stents. In older patients with pulmonary atresia and ventricular septal defect repeat cardiac catheterization and angiography is the only precise means of evaluating the pulmonary circulation with any degree of certainty. In addition, it permits further transcatheter interventions to be performed, e.g. coil embolization of collaterals should that be necessary.

In patients with pulmonary atresia and intact ventricular septum the need for cardiac catheterization is governed by the anatomy, coronary artery anomalies and, most importantly, to assess the impact of the many staged surgical interventions that these patients undergo.

Surgery

In patients with pulmonary atresia and ventricular septal defect major surgical goals are:

1. closure of the ventricular septal defect;
2. establishing continuity between the right ventricle and pulmonary arteries;
3. elimination of excessive collateral circulation.

Depending on the site of atresia of the right ventricular outflow tract it may be possible to open and enlarge the pulmonary annulus with a transannular patch. However, a conduit between the right ventricle and pulmonary artery will usually be required. If there is free flow of blood from the right ventricle to pulmonary artery, it may then be possible to close the ventricular septal defect. However, if this results in right ventricular hypertension, a fenestration can be placed in the ventricular patch. The presence of MAPCAS present a major surgical challenge. The aim is to 'unifocalize' the pulmonary blood supply connecting the MAPCAS to the central pulmonary arteries, followed by connection to the right ventricle. In some, this can easily be achieved if the central pulmonary arteries are of an adequate size and most of the lung has dual blood supply. In these cases it may be possible to ligate the MAPCAS or embolize them at cardiac catheterization prior to surgical intervention. Surgery may not be feasible in patients with severe hypoplasia of the central pulmonary arteries, multiple peripheral pulmonary arterial stenoses together with large MAPCAS. If these patients are haemo-dynamically well-balanced with an acceptable quality of life and exercise toler-ance, they are best left alone. However, should there be clinical deterioration or progessive severe cyanosis with its concomitant problems, it may be possible to increase pulmonary blood flow by shunting procedures or relieve severe stenoses in the MAPCAS by balloon dilatation with stent implantation. The majority of patients with pulmonary atresia and ventricular septal defect who have under-gone attempted correction will require further surgery as the development of conduit obstruction is almost inevitable. The site of the conduit just beneath the sternum will require careful consideration as to the means of establishing cardiopulmonary bypass prior to attempted replacement (see Chapter 20).

The timing and the type of surgical intervention is dictated by the patients' clinical condition. On the one hand those presenting in the neonatal period with severe cyanosis may undergo a shunt procedure if the pulmonary arteries are of adequate size. Alternatively, those presenting with severe breathlessness may require coil embolization or surgical ligation of collaterals. The timing of attempted correction depends on the experience of the local unit. Some argue that the sooner continuity is established between the right ventricle and the pulmonary artery with the free egress of blood from right ventricle to pulmonary artery the better. However, this will necessitate surgical revision of the conduit in early childhood.

Patients with pulmonary atresia and intact ventricular septum present a different dilemma. As stated above ductal patency is essential for survival in the neonatal period. With closure of the duct, the patient dies. The type of surgery depends on the size of the right ventricle and the presence or absence of right ventricular dependent coronary artery circulation. In some patients with an adequate sized right ventricle and no major right ventricular coronary artery fistulae it may be possible to perform laser or radiofrequency pulmonary valvotomy followed by pulmonary valvoplasty at cardiac catheterization. Although feasible it obviously depends to some extent on the length of atresia. Alternatively, a shunt such as a modified Blalock Taussig shunt may augment pulmonary blood supply and ensure survival beyond infancy. It is clear in some patients that the right ventricle is too small to be considered for future biventricular repair and some form of Fontan circulation needs to be considered. At one extreme are a subset of patients with severe hypoplasia of the right ventricular dependent coronary circulation in whom conventional surgery may have little to offer. Cardiac transplantation may be the only alternative. In patients with right ventricular dependent coronary circulation the establishment of right ventricular to pulmonary artery continuity is based on the premiss that right ventricular decompression will not compromise the coronary circulation and lead to myocardial ischaemia. Precise preoperative information is essential and the management of these patients should be left to the tertiary referral centre.

Long-term follow-up

Pulmonary atresia with intact ventricular septum

There are very few adult survivors of early palliation. Although several small studies have shown that the right ventricle can increases in size after palliation, abnormalities of right ventricular function are always present after biventricular repair. Although systolic function may be well-preserved there is usually evidence of restrictive right ventricular physiology. None the less, these patients can lead relatively normal lives. Some patients have a univentricular repair or Fontan procedure (see Chapter 10). Follow-up in this group is similar to those of the Fontan group as a whole.

Pulmonary atresia with VSD

In patients with good sized confluent pulmonary arteries who have been well palliated, complete repair with a RV to PA conduit should be possible with relatively low risk. Their follow-up statistics and problems are similar to those with tetralogy of Fallot. In the remainder, survival depends on the adequacy of pulmonary blood supply and the success of palliative surgery. Many surgical strategies have been proposed and many patients have died as a result of well-intentioned radical palliative surgery with insertion of conduits, pericardial tubes, shunts, etc. Results of this type of surgery are improving and should be pursued in some centres. None the less for some patients with haemodynamically balanced multifocal pulmonary blood supply, no surgery may be the best option, with a view ultimately to cardiopulmonary transplantation. In general terms, aortic regurgitation must be looked for during follow-up, and although ventricular arrhythmias do not appear to be as common in patients who have undergone surgery for pulmonary atresia and ventricular septal defect as in their counterparts with classical tetralogy of Fallot, any symptoms of presyncope or syncope should be taken seriously.

Conclusions

1. There are relatively few long-term survivors with pulmonary atresia with intact septum although complete biventricular repair or conversion to a Fontan circulation is increasingly successfully when performed in childhood.
2. Some cases of pulmonary atresia with ventricular septal defect are managed identically to that of 'simple' tetralogy of Fallot, although a right ventricle to pulmonary artery conduit of some kind is more frequently required.
3. 'Complex' pulmonary atresia (with multiple aortopulmonary collateral arteries) has a relatively poor prognosis. However, some patients remain relatively well for many years without surgical intervention.

Key references

de Leval M, Bull C, Hopkins R et al (1985) Decision-making in the definitive repair of the heart with a small right ventricle. *Circulation* **72** (suppl. II): 52–60.

Puga FJ, Leoni FE, Julsrud PR et al (1989) Complete repair of pulmonary atresia, ventricular septal defect and severe peripheral arborization abnormalities of the central pulmonary arteries: Experience with preliminary unifocalisation procedures in 38 patients. *J Thorac Cardiovasc Surg* **98**: 1018–28.

10 Univentricular Atrioventricular Connection and the Fontan Procedure

Introduction

To the unfamiliar this term could be a little threatening. In fact, it merely groups together a 'family' of conditions which are characterized by the presence of one dominant and useful ventricular chamber (formerly 'single ventricle', 'primitive ventricle'). The ventricular mass rarely consists of a single ventricle however, there usually being a second small and 'rudimentary' ventricle. This has little or no significance in terms of pump function, but is highly significant in terms of both diagnostic morphology and the arterial connections to it. The term is also a useful one in that the clinical management of these patients, despite widely disparate atrial and ventricular anatomy, follows broadly similar lines ultimately directed towards a univentricular 'correction' or Fontan-like procedure.

Key anatomical features

These hearts are characterized by the majority of the atrial mass being connected predominantly to one of the ventricles. The mode of atrioventricular connection varies widely however. The two major diagnostic groups are absent right atrioventricular connection (tricuspid atresia) and double inlet ventricle.

Absent right connection (tricuspid atresia)

The term absent connection is more morphologically correct than that of the usual 'tricuspid atresia' because, other than in exceptional cases, there is no tricuspid valve tissue in these hearts. Indeed, there is no potential communication between the right atrium and the ventricular mass, the floor of the right atrium being an infolding of the walls of the right atrium and underlying ventricle. The only exit from the right atrium is through the atrial septum, all the systemic and pulmonary venous return entering the left atrium and then the left ventricle via a single left atrioventricular valve. As a result the left ventricle is large and 'dominant' and the right ventricle is small and 'rudimentary'. The ventriculoarterial connection is usually concordant (classical tricuspid atresia) with the aorta arising from the left ventricle and the pulmonary arteries arising from the right ventricle. There is usually a ventricular septal defect which allows antegrade flow from the left ventricle, through the right ventricle, to the pulmonary artery. This is usually small and restrictive however, and for this reason the pulmonary arteries are often small and pulmonary blood flow limited. In approximately 15% the ventriculoarterial connection is discordant (transposition of the great arteries), although this proportion is considerably lower in late survivors with tricuspid atresia. This is because it is the systemic blood flow which is often restricted in these patients with consequent hypoplasia of the aorta and arch, complicating considerably their management. For brevity, only the commoner forms of absent connection have been described, but it should be remembered that absent left atrioventricular connection may some-times be encountered and that the morphology of the ventricular mass and the ventriculoarterial connection is independent of the atrial and junctional anatomy, all combinations having been described.

Double inlet ventricle

The term univentricular atrioventricular connection applies to these hearts because both atria are completely or predominantly connected to the dominant ventricle usually via two separate atrioventricular valves (Figure 1). When there is a common atrioventricular valve the 75% rule applies, more than three-quarters of the valve and junction needing to be committed to the dominant ventricle. This definition does not, of course, exclude the possibility of straddling valve tissue with chordal attachments of the atrioventricular valve in both ventricles, and again is independent of atrial and ventricular anatomy and ventriculoarterial connection. None the less, some types are more commonly seen than others. Double inlet left ventricle with a discordant ventriculoarterial connection, the aorta arising from an anterior right or left sided rudimentary right ventricle, is commonly encountered. It is the size and anatomy of the ventricular septal defect (VSD) which is critical to the presentation and management of these patients. If small, the VSD will limit systemic blood flow and aortic arch anomalies are thus common. Furthermore, unless there is subpulmonary or pulmonary valve stenosis, there will be unlimited pulmonary blood flow and ultimately pulmonary vascular disease will develop, if left. Occasionally a 'balanced' pulmonary blood flow will result from 'just enough' limitation of pulmonary blood flow and some of these patients will survive unoperated into adult life, without the development of pulmonary vascular disease. This is particularly the case if there is a concordant ventriculoarterial connection (Holmes heart). Double inlet right ventricle is more unusual,

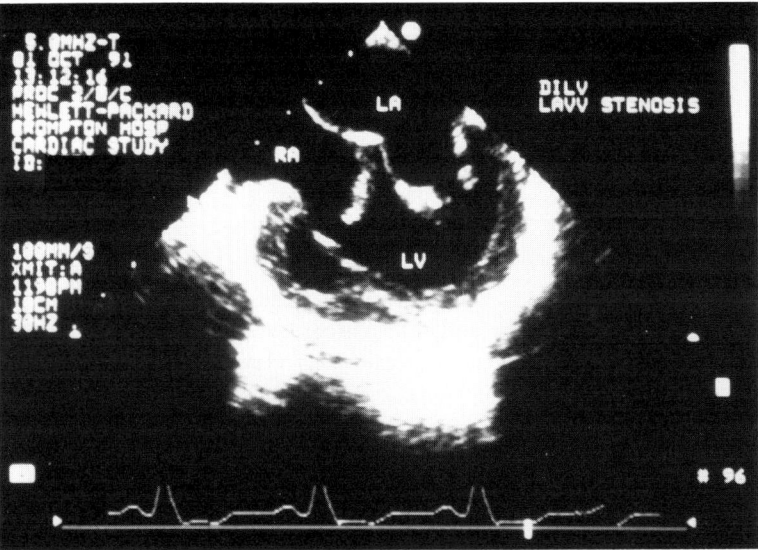

Figure 1. Transoesophageal echocardiogram from a patient with two seperate atrioventricular valves entering a large left ventricle (Double inlet left ventricle). In this case there is a stenotic left atrioventricular valve with left atrial hypertension. RA, right atrium; LA, left atrium; LV, left ventricle.

accounting for only 20% of double inlet ventricles. More often than in double inlet left, there is a common atrioventricular valve. The small rudimentary posterior left ventricle may lack a well-developed inlet and outlet (other than a VSD) the commonest ventriculoarterial connection being double outlet right ventricle.

Management

These patients have conditions amongst the most complex of all congenital heart disease and subsequently the case notes of an adult may be almost incomprehensible, with multiple and varied diagnoses, multiple palliative procedures and contradictory results from previous cardiac catheterizations. Conversely, some patients with limited but 'balanced' pulmonary blood flow remain virtually asymptomatic and not inconsiderable numbers survive unoperated into adult life. There are also increasing numbers of older patients who have undergone 'definite palliation' in the form of a Fontan procedure, or one of its variants. All in all this group represents one of the most challenging, in terms of their investigation and management and their care should be restricted to special centres.

Early palliation

Limited pulmonary blood flow

Most patients with classical tricuspid atresia will have undergone surgery to increase their pulmonary blood flow. Modified Blalock Taussig, classical Blalock, Waterston and Potts Shunts have all been performed. The latter three require care during subsequent investigations. A prerequisite for success of Fontan procedure and other venopulmonary connections (see below) is a low pulmonary vascular resistance and minor degrees of even unilateral pulmonary vascular damage, which is not uncommon after classical Blalock, Waterston and Potts Shunts, will increase the morbidity and mortality of atriopulmonary or venopulmonary anastomosis. Some degree of ventricular volume overload is inevitable after any of these shunts, even when providing perfect palliation. Their potential long-term adverse effects with atrioventricular valve regurgitation and ventricular failure has led to the development of several direct venopulmonary and atriopulmonary operations. By diverting systemic venous blood into the pulmonary arteries the ventricular volume load is reduced, and oxygenation is more efficient. The pulmonary blood flow is essentially 'pumpless' after these procedures (see below) which is why success is dependent on the pulmonary vascular resistance being low (ideally less than 2 Wood Units). There are two 'partial' procedures:

Classical Glenn procedure

This very successful procedure is now only rarely performed. It is performed via a left thoracotomy and consists of an end-to-end anastomosis between the superior caval vein and the right pulmonary artery. Blood flow to the left lung is usually antegradely from the ventricle, or occasionally via a left sided aortopulmonary shunt. First performed in the 1950s there is now over 30-year follow-up in these patients. It has proved to be remarkably successful, with a low operative and late mortality and good palliation of cyanosis in many. Its reputation has been tarnished however, by the relatively high incidence (up to 70%) of acquired pulmonary arteriovenous fistulae in the right lung with recurrence of, or increasing, cyanosis. The reason for their development is unknown, and their importance is perhaps overemphasized. None the less, this complication should be considered in any patient with worsening cyanosis. The diagnosis is relatively simply using cross-sectional echocardiography. In the absence of another connection between the superior caval vein and pulmonary venous atrium, an injection of an echocardiographic contrast agent into a vein in the right arm will demonstrate filling of the pulmonary venous atrium after a few seconds of passage through the lungs, via the fistulae. Their treatment is less easy. Coil embolization may be appropriate if localized and discrete, but often the whole of the right lung (or more usually its lower lobe) is abnormal (Figure 2). There is

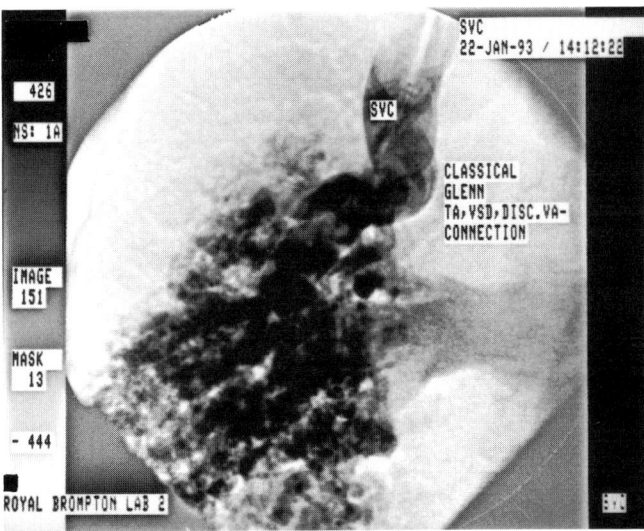

Figure 2. Aquired pulmonary arteriovenous fistulae of the lung after a Classical Glenn procedure (see text for details). Injection into the superior caval vein (SVC) fills the right lower lobe which has a diffusely abnormal vasculature due to the development of fistulae. Note how the pulmonary veins have filled very early.

some anecdotal evidence that conversion to a complete Fontan procedure leads to regression of the fistulae, but this remains experimental.

Bidirectional Glenn procedure

This operation has gained popularity over the past five years or so. Its advantage, as the name suggests, is that the pulmonary arteries are left in continuity. It is usually performed via a median sternotomy, the superior caval vein being anastomosed end-to-side to the pulmonary artery. It is particularly successful in small children, in whom the resulting arterial oxygen saturation may be as high as 85–90%. The resulting arterial oxygen saturation tends to be lower in older children and adults. The difference almost certainly reflects the relatively larger venous return from the upper body in smaller children compared with adults. Indeed, our experience is that the bidirectional Glenn procedure provides for unsatisfactory arterial oxygenation when it is the sole source of pulmonary blood flow in adults. As a prelude to the Fontan procedure it remains a useful procedure in young children however.

Increased pulmonary blood flow

In patients with double inlet left ventricle and tricuspid atresia with ventriculo-arterial discordance the pulmonary artery arises from the dominant chamber.

Unless there is coexisting subpulmonary or pulmonary valve stenosis, pulmonary blood flow is unlimited and pulmonary vascular disease will rapidly develop. These patients require early and effective banding of the pulmonary artery to protect the pulmonary vascular bed from damage. As a result, few patients will escape further surgery in their early years, as they 'outgrow' their band. A significant proportion of these patients present with or develop impaired systemic blood flow. Blood flow to the aorta is via a ventricular septal defect and the rudimentary right ventricle. If either is restrictive there will effectively be 'subaortic' stenosis which in turn leads to systemic ventricular hypertrophy, in itself a risk factor for the Fontan procedure (see below). In infants presenting with coarctation or interruption of the aorta, the outlook has been particularly bleak, with very few late survivors. Increasing awareness of the importance of subaortic restriction and the development of left ventricular hypertrophy has improved the prognosis and led to the development of several strategies to improve systemic blood flow, all of which are appropriate in later life: there are two approaches:

1. Direct enlargement of the ventricular septal defect.
2. Creation of an aortopulmonary connection: Aortopulmonary window or end-to-side pulmonary artery-to-aorta connection (Damus-Kaye-Stanzl procedure).

Such is the importance of even a minor degree of subaortic stenosis, that it should be excluded in all patients with suspicious underlying anatomy. A resting, exercise or isoprenaline-induced gradient between left ventricle and aorta will almost certainly worsen with time or after the Fontan procedure and should be relieved.

The Fontan procedure

The ultimate goal for patients with a univentricular atrioventricular connection is a Fontan procedure or one of its variants. It was first described as a definitive treatment for tricuspid atresia but since then its indications, preoperative criteria, and surgical technique have all evolved. An understanding of this evolution is necessary however, as many of the patients operated upon in the 1970s and 1980s are now entering adult life.

A brief history of the Fontan procedure

Fontan and Choussat originally described their atriopulmonary connection in 1973. It is now known that neither the atrium nor inlet or outlet valves are necessary, and indeed may be disadvantageous under some circumstances. The Kreutzer modification introduced the direct atriopulmonary anastomosis without valves and its indications subsequently widened to include patients with double inlet ventricle (combined with patch closure of the right atrioventricular valve and closure of any atrial septal defect). The Kawashima procedure or total cavopulmonary shunt was first described for the treatment of patients with complex venous and atrial anatomy. In those with azygous continuation to a superior caval vein, connection of the caval vein directly diverts all but the hepatic venous drainage into the pulmonary arteries. Despite the lack of the 'atrial pump' this procedure carries a low mortality and gives an excellent functional result in carefully selected patients. It is more important in a broader sense as it illustrated that atrial contraction was not fundamental to the success of these procedures and subsequently the total cavopulmonary anastomosis (bi-directional Glenn procedure with intra-atrial baffle of the inferior caval vein to the pulmonary artery) has become established as the procedure of first choice for all patients other than those with tricuspid atresia.

Finally, the concept of the partial or fenestrated Fontan was introduced. This approach was developed in response to the unacceptably high early mortality (up to 30% in some groups) and morbidity for the high risk candidate. By leaving an inter-atrial communication the systemic venous system is 'decompressed' and the systemic cardiac output is augmented. This is at the expense of residual cyanosis of course, but the communication can subsequently be closed by tightening a subcutaneous snare left around the defect or by transvenous umbrella placement, days or weeks after the procedure. This simple modification has substantially reduced early mortality and morbidity.

Selection/risk factors

Some of the 'Ten Commandments' of Choussat and Fontan are now known to be less important. There are three main risk factors for poor outcome:

1. Raised preoperative pulmonary vascular resistance (>4 Wood Units) and/or raised pulmonary arterial pressure (mean >15 mmHg).
2. Age less than 2 years or greater than 14 years.
3. The presence of ventricular hypertrophy.

Other haemodynamic abnormalities, e.g. severe ventricular dysfunction, atrio-ventricular valve regurgitation, pulmonary artery distortion, are also clearly important and to some extent decision-making has to be individualized, particularly in older children and adults in whom surgery is often truly 'elective'.

Follow-up of the post Fontan patient

The functional outcome of the Fontan procedure ranges from virtual normality with no symptoms to severe disability with exercise limitation, recurrent pleural

effusions and ascites and early death. The key point to remember is the remark-
able lack of 'reserve' in the circulation so that even minor changes in haemodynamic status can lead to rapid conversion of the former to the latter. There is no
place for the wait-and-see approach in these patients. Significant deterioration
requires careful reassessment and early referral for specialist treatment.

Clinical assessment

Following a successful complete atriopulmonary or cavopulmonary connection
the patients should be pink and fully saturated. Arterial desaturation implies a
residual shunt either intracardiac, intrapulmonary (see above) or occasionally due
to opening of abnormal venous connections allowing a right-to-left shunt.
Pulsatility of a small liver or an obvious 'a' wave in a modestly elevated jugular
venous pressure is expected after atriopulmonary anastomosis because of retrograde flow in the great veins. Indeed, the central venous pressure is always
elevated but gross hepatomegaly, peripheral oedema, ascites or evidence of
pleural effusion, and importantly the late development of any of these signs,
are abnormal and require investigation. The heart sounds are usually quiet, the
second sound most often being single. The Fontan circuit does not generate
murmurs even when severely obstructed. A loud ejection murmur with a carotid
thrill should raise the suspicion of subaortic obstruction and pansystolic murmur
implies either systemic atrioventricular valve regurgitation or occasionally a
leaking patch over an excluded right atrioventricular valve in double inlet left
ventricle for example. The latter is rarely haemodynamically significant but a
useful sign of a large patch leak is the presence of a large or dominant v-wave on
a jugular venous pulse recording.

Electrocardiogram

This is rarely helpful in assessing the haemodynamic result. Right atrial hypertrophy will be seen in those with an atriopulmonary connection and ventricular
hypertrophy and dominance will go along with the morphology of dominant
ventricle.

Chest Radiograph

Cardiomegaly is usually related to dilatation of the right atrium, which may be
massive. The pulmonary vascular markings are normal or decreased, reflecting a
slightly low resting cardiac output. Increased pulmonary vascular markings on
the routine film usually imply a residual shunt as pulmonary venous congestion is
extremely poorly tolerated and patients with a raised left atrial pressure will be
very unwell.

Cross-sectional echocardiography

The right atrium is usually larger than normal and the atrial septum will bow from right to left after atriopulmonary anastomosis. Similarly, the coronary sinus may be markedly enlarged if incorporated on the systemic venous side of the circulation. The intra-atrial baffle of the total cavopulmonary connection is more difficult to image in its entirety. A particularly difficult area is the anastomosis of its upper end to the underside of the transected superior caval vein (which itself is anastomosed to the underside of the pulmonary artery). Longitudinal-plane transoesophageal echocardiography is particularly useful when assessing the Fontan circulation, particularly the cavopulmonary connections. Although either or both the transthoracic or transoesophageal approach may demonstrate the distal atriopulmonary (Figure 3) or cavopulmonary connection, sometimes it is impossible to exclude obstruction using imaging alone. Doppler flow studies are particularly useful in this regard. There will be a marked respiratory variation in flow velocities with respiration (particularly following cavopulmonary anastomosis) but any velocity in excess of 1.5 metres per second or significant turbulence demonstrated by colour flow mapping deserves further investigation. Systemic ventricular inflow may also show marked respiratory variation. Incoordinate relaxation is a feature of these ventricles and so a prolonged isovolumic relaxation period, diminished early rapid filling and dominant atrial systolic filling is seen frequently. Systolic ventricular performance is usually within normal limits.

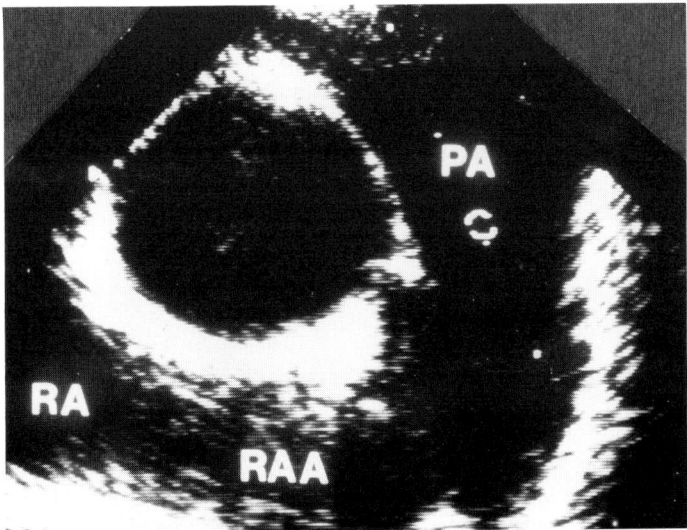

Figure 3. Transoesophageal echocardiogram from a patient after the Fontan procedure. The right atrium (RA) has been connected to the pulmonary artery (PA) via the right atrial appendage (RAA). None of these features were demonstrated using conventional transthoracic imaging.

Magnetic resonance imaging

This is one of the situations where MRI may be very useful, particularly if velocity mapping is available. MRI should show the venous connections and peripheral pulmonary arterial anatomy well, but if there remains any doubt regarding possible obstruction then cardiac catheterization will be required.

Cardiac catheterization

Because even minor degrees of obstruction have such sinister prognostic and functional implications, cardiac catheterization should be performed in any patient in whom doubt remains after non-invasive studies. Remember a mean gradient of 1–2 mmHg may be a significant gradient in this sluggish, low-flow circulation. The commonest sites of obstruction are at the anastomotic line between atrium and pulmonary artery (particularly if a valved conduit has been used), and at the origin of the pulmonary arteries. Balloon dilatation and stent implantation are highly successful and particularly beneficial when the high risk of reoperation is taken into account.

Late problems

It is too early in the evolution of the total cavopulmonary anastomosis to discuss late complications. It is hoped the intra-atrial baffle will avoid over-distention of the atrium and so avoid some of the problems of the atriopulmonary anastomosis. It is itself however a more complex procedure with many more anastomotic lines and more liberal use of artificial material and only time will tell whether it is a better alternative. The atriopulmonary anastomosis has several late problems, all of which are to some extent inter-related:

1. Pathway obstruction.
2. Arrhythmias.
3. Thromboembolism.
4. Congestive cardiac failure.

Pathway obstruction

The importance of this has already been emphasized, but bears repeating. The cardiac output after these procedures depends on the modest pressure gradient between the pulmonary artery and left atrium. Thus even minor degrees of obstruction can substantially reduce cardiac output, lead to a dilated right atrium, and increase the likelihood of arrhythmia and atrial clot formation because of stasis. Reoperation for any reason carries a high mortality in these patients but thankfully balloon dilatation with or without stent replacement will relieve all but the most resistant stenoses.

Arrhythmias

Not surprisingly, atrial arrhythmias are quite common after atriopulmonary anastomosis. Bradycardias are usually well tolerated but tachyarrhythmias may be life threatening. When presenting as a new symptom, pathway obstruction must be ruled out, and the presence of intra-atrial thrombus excluded. Atrial flutter is the commonest arrhythmia and is perhaps best converted to sinus rhythm by DC cardioversion or transvenous atrioversion. Prophylactic drug therapy varies in its efficacy; sometimes this arrhythmia is remarkably resistant and multiple therapy may be required. Atrial fibrillation is similarly difficult to prevent and ultimately suppression of ventricular rate may be the only thera-peutic option, albeit frequently with a much reduced exercise tolerance. The role of conversion to a cavopulmonary connection (to decompress the atrium and so reduce the stimulus to arrhythmia) is unknown.

Thromboembolism

All patients with chronic arrhythmia, stents or unrelieved obstruction should be formally anticoagulated. The incidence of covert asymptomatic thromboembo-lism is unknown but recent studies using transoesophageal and intravascular ultrasound suggest a worryingly high incidence of atrial and intrapulmonary thrombosis (Figure 4). Assuming there are no contraindications it is our policy to recommend anticoagulation to all patients after the Fontan procedure, although admittedly there are no data to support this.

Congestive cardiac failure (death)

There is an ongoing attrition after the Fontan procedure, with the late mortality approaching 25% at 15 years follow-up. Reoperation, overt thrombosis and arrhythmia are all associated with poor outcome, but some develop a progres-sively worsening cardiac output which is largely unexplained. A rising central venous pressure will lead to the development of pleural effusion, ascites and peripheral oedema and a vicious cycle can rapidly become established. The development of protein losing enteropathy (at least in part related to the raised CVP) is notoriously difficult to treat other than symptomatically with protein replacement infusions and indicates a poor prognosis. Some will respond to diuretic therapy but over-dehydration will simply lower the cardiac output still further. It is rare that a patient with unexplained severe deterioration responds to

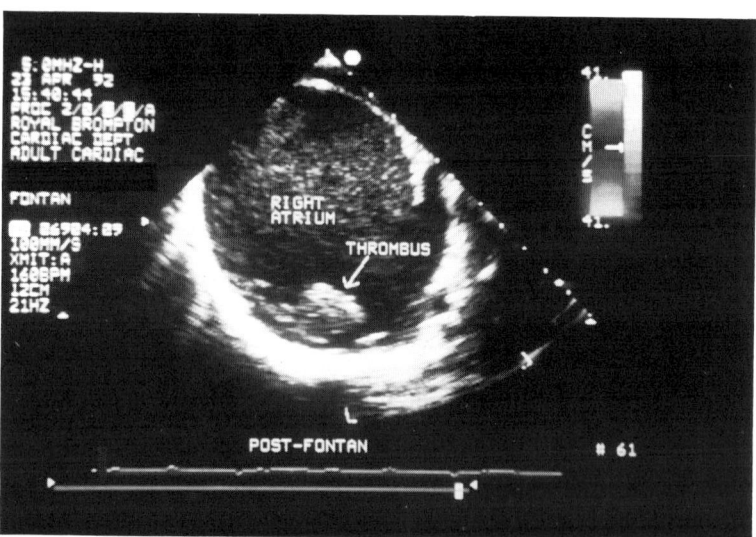

Figure 4. Transoesophageal ultrasound scan showing an occult mural thrombus in a patient with a stenosed right atrial to pulmonary artery connection. Note also the 'spontaneous' contrast in the atrium.

medical therapy and early assessment for cardiac transplantation may be the best option.

Key references

Deanfield J (1991) Arrhythmias after the Fontan procedure. *Circulation* **84** (suppl. III); 162–67.

de Leval MR, Kilner P, Gewellig M, Bull C (1988) Total cavopulmonary connection: A logical alternative to atriopulmonary connection for complex Fontan operations. *J Thorac Cardiovasc Surg* **96**: 682–95.

Fontan F, Baudet E (1971) Surgical repair of tricuspid atresia. *Thorax* **26**: 240–48.

Fontan F, Kirklin JW, Fernandezt et al (1990) Outcome after a 'perfect' Fontan operation. *Circulation* **81**: 1520–36.

Humes RA, Mair DD, Porter CBJ et al (1988) Results of modified Fontan operation in adults. *Am J Cardiol* **61**: 602–04.

Mazzera E, Corno A, Picardo S et al (1989) Bidirectional cavopulmonary shunts: Clinical applications as staged or definitive palliation. *Ann Thorac Surg* **47**: 415–20.

Non-cyanotic heart disease

11 Atrial Septal Defect

In collaboration with SJD Brecker

Introduction

The interatrial septal defect is the most commonly encountered, previously undetected, form of congenital heart disease seen in the adult patient. Ventricular septal defects are more common in the paediatric age group but many will close spontaneously or be detected and repaired. By contrast, the atrial septal defect will often go unrecognized until it is responsible for symptoms or a complication such as a paradoxical embolus in adult life. Overall it comprises 7% of all congenital heart disease and approximately 30% of that in an adult population.

Key anatomical features

The defects are defined based upon the portion of the atrial septum which is deficient – thus the **ostium secumdum** defect, accounting for 70% of defects, is due to an absence of septal tissue in the region of the oval fossa, and is usually 1–2 cm in diameter. They are quite different to the patent foramen ovale which is a flap like slit without true deficiency of the septum. Defects of the superior **sinus venosus** type (15% of total) are located at the mouth of the superior vena cava, high in the atrial septum such that the superior caval vein overrides the septum (Figure 2, Chapter 3). This is often associated with anomalous drainage of the right sided pulmonary veins. Inferior sinus venosus defects open at the mouth of the inferior caval vein and although extremely rare are a cause of undiagnosed cyanosis in adults. The **ostium primum** defect describes the atrial component to the spectrum of lesions described as **atrioventricular septal defects**. The atrioventricular septal defects comprise the range of malformations that are manifestations of the absence of the atrioventricular septum. They are unified by the presence of a common atrioventricular junction, and abnormal atrioventricular valve anatomy. The simple ostium primum defect (or 'partial atrioventricular septal defect') is characterized by a large interatrial defect inferior to the lower end of the atrial septum but with no direct ventricular communication. The left atrioventricular valve is not a true 'mitral' valve because it has three leaflets, and may therefore be regurgitant. The 'complete atrioventricular septal defect' (or 'common atrioventricular canal'), in addition to the interatrial communication, includes an inlet ventricular septal defect and usually a common atrioventricular valve. The common atrioventricular valve characteristically has five leaflets including superior and inferior bridging leaflets (bridging the crest of the ventricular septum). In both partial and complete forms, the left ventricular outflow tract is elongated ('goose-neck' deformity). Because of the proximity of the defect to the conducting system, abnormalities of atrioventricular conduction are frequently present.

Pathophysiology

The basic physiology of all types of atrial septal defect is shunting of blood from left to right. The degree of the shunt will depend upon the size of the defect, the relative compliance of the right and left ventricles and the relative pulmonary and systemic vascular resistances. The left to right shunt will thus increase the volume load of the right atrium and ventricle which will become dilated. Pulmonary blood flow will be increased and the pulmonary arteries and veins will become enlarged. In all cases some shunting will occur from right to left and this fact may be used in diagnosis using a systemic venous bubble contrast injection. On echocardiography bubbles may be seen in the left heart. A characteristic finding in inferior sinus venosus defects is the much more marked right-to-left shunting of bubbles when injected into the lower body, than when injected into the arm. During early life, the pulmonary vascular bed is able to cope with the increased flow, and pulmonary vascular resistance is normal. In a proportion of patients with both secundum and primum defects (approximately 10% of both) and large shunts, pulmonary vascular disease and pulmonary hypertension develop. As it does so, the size of the shunt decreases, probably related to reduced right ventricular compliance. Eventually the shunt will become predominantly right to left, and cyanosis ensues (the Eisenmenger syndrome).

Clinical findings

Symptoms

Ostium secundum defect

Patients are often asymptomatic in early life although close questioning of a young adult may reveal some evidence of exercise intolerance. In any event, symptoms increase with age such that over 70% of adults will be symptomatic by 40 years. Symptoms will include palpitation due to atrial arrhythmias, exertional dyspnoea and fatigue, a productive cough and recurrent chest infections, ankle swelling related to the development of right ventricular disease and symptoms of paradoxical emboli. Chest pain similar to angina may occur and may be related to right ventricular ischaemia. It is important to remember that patients may develop ischaemic and hypertensive heart disease in addition, and these features may complicate the clinical picture. By the sixth decade virtually all patients will have symptoms.

Ostium primum defect

Symptoms will be as for the secundum defect but will be more severe if there is associated left atrioventricular valve regurgitation. There are also the added complications of syncope due to heart block, and propensity to infective endocarditis.

Signs

Ostium secundum defect

The pulse will be normal or small volume, and the jugular venous pressure normal or raised if there is pulmonary hypertension or right ventricular disease. The right ventricular impulse will be prominent, and on auscultation, the first sound will be loud and the second will be fixed and widely split in inspiration and expiration. An ejection systolic flow murmur in the pulmonary area and a mid-diastolic tricuspid flow murmur are present and related to increased right sided flows.

Ostium primum defect

The physical signs will be as for the secundum defect, usually with the added feature of a pansystolic murmur at the apex related to left atrioventricular valve regurgitation. The physical signs of pulmonary hypertension may be present in both secundum and primum defects: palpable and sustained right ventricular impulse related to right ventricular hypertrophy, palpable and loud pulmonary closure component to the second heart sound, a right sided fourth heart sound, a tricuspid regurgitant murmur, a pulmonary ejection click and the early diastolic murmur of pulmonary regurgitation. If shunt reversal and the Eisenmenger syndrome has developed, then central cyanosis and clubbing will be present, together with a low volume pulse, and the signs of pulmonary hypertension and right ventricular disease.

Investigations

Electrocardiogram

Ostium secundum defect

Partial or complete right bundle branch block is present predominantly due to the enlargement of the right ventricle, together with right axis deviation. The PR interval may prolong with increasing age.

Ostium primum defect

Because of the proximity of the defect edges to the atrioventricular node and bundle of His, the performance of both may be disturbed. Prolongation of the PR interval is common, and right bundle branch block is usually present. Delayed activation of the left anterior fascicle occurs because of the disturbed anatomy of the bundle of His, and striking left axis deviation is present in the majority. Right ventricular hypertrophy with a strain pattern in V_1 and V_2 suggests pulmonary hypertension.

Chest X-ray

In both secundum and primum defects there will be moderate cardiac enlargement related to dilatation of right-sided chambers, a small aortic knuckle, a large main pulmonary artery and pulmonary plethora. As pulmonary hypertension ensues, peripheral pruning of the pulmonary vasculature occurs.

Echocardiography

Transthoracic echocardiography identifies the precise anatomy in the majority of cases and contrast studies will reveal shunting. The right atrium and ventricle will be dilated, and paradoxical septal motion may be present. Features of pulmonary hypertension may be present, and the peak right ventricular – right atrial pressure drop can be estimated on Doppler echocardiography. For sinus venosus defects, longitudinal plane transoesophageal echocardiography may demonstrate the defect extremely well (Figure 2, Chapter 3). Echocardiography of the ostium primum defect should clarify the nature of the atrioventricular connection, the characteristic bridging leaflets of the common atrioventricular valve and any associated mitral valve abnormalities. It is worth noting that commonly there is a recess beneath the superior bridging leaflet, when seen in the apical four-chamber view. This can sometimes be mistaken as a ventricular septal defect, but this can be excluded by careful Doppler studies. Doppler echocardiography can also be used to obtain pulsed Doppler flow velocity integrals of aortic (systemic) and pulmonary forward flow, and in this way a useful estimate of the shunt can be obtained.

Cardiac catheterization

Echocardiography has now made this an obsolete way of investigating atrial septal defects, although catheterization may still be performed to assess the shunt using saturation data. It is usually easy to cross the defect from the femoral approach, and to enter all pulmonary veins. Measurement of pulmonary artery pressures and cardiac outputs may be required to estimate pulmonary vascular resistance in patients being considered for surgical repair or heart–lung transplantation.

Natural history

Ostium secundum defect

These defects may remain undetected in early childhood, and although a small proportion of infants will have congestive heart failure, the rule is for most children and adolescents to lead a normal life. Nevertheless it is well-recognized that after surgical repair the patient may recognize a greater exercise tolerance than previously. The symptoms described above develop in adult life such that by 40 most individuals will be symptomatic. Atrial arrhythmias (fibrillation and flutter) develop progressively with age, and there is little evidence that late surgical correction prevents their development. Pulmonary vascular disease develops in approximately 10%, and usually appears between the ages of 20 and 40 years. The reasons for the development of pulmonary hypertension in some but not others with this defect remain obscure, but the complication is more common in women, and living at high altitude may predispose to premature pulmonary vascular disease. Without significant pulmonary hypertension, survival to old age is possible. However, the development of pulmonary vascular disease markedly reduces life expectancy with most patients dying before the sixth decade. Previous studies reveal a low overall mortality rate in the first two decades (below 1%), rising to 3% in the third decade and to 7.5% in the sixth.

Ostium primum defect

In the preoperative era, the average life expectancy of patients with an unrepaired primum defect was 30 years. The natural history of a partial atrioventricular

septal defect without much mitral regurgitation is similar to that of a large
secundum defect. Once again pulmonary vascular disease develops in a minority
and symptomatic deterioration with atrial arrhythmias is similar to the secundum
defect. The natural history of the ostium primum defect in general however, is
less good than the secundum defect because of abnormalities of the atrioventricular valves (mitral regurgitation most commonly) and the conduction system.
Significant mitral regurgitation increases the left-to-right shunt and moderate
pulmonary hypertension develops.

Pregnancy

This is usually well-tolerated in uncomplicated atrial septal defects. However
significant pulmonary hypertension is associated with increased maternal and
fetal morbidity and mortality, and pregnancy should be avoided in the Eisenmenger state (see Chapter 22). Rapidly progressive pulmonary vascular disease
can develop in pregnancy, and thus routine closure prior to pregnancy is
recommended.

Management of the adult with ASD: to close or not to close

Ostium secundum defects

Most children will have undergone routine closure of their atrial septal defect if
discovered before adolescence, provided it is of haemodynamic significance
(pulmonary:systemic flow ratio of greater than 1.5:1) and pulmonary vascular
resistance is normal. This is performed for prophylactic reasons: to prevent the
development of pulmonary vascular disease, right ventricular failure and paradoxical emboli. Closure in the older patient is a more contentious topic. Most
agree that in the young adult with symptoms and normal pulmonary vascular
resistance, closure is recommended for the reasons stated above, and in females,
to prevent potential complications of pregnancy. The surgical risk is low (<1%)
in such patients, and interventional techniques using clamshells and umbrellas
may obviate the need for surgery. Similarly, adults with an episode of paradoxical
embolus should have their defect closed. In adults between the ages of 20 to 50
years the indications for closure are less clear, and in those with additional
hypertensive or ischaemic left ventricular disease, operative morbidity and
mortality are higher and long-term benefits less well proven. Interventional
device closure carries lower risks and may be performed when technically
feasible.

In patients over the age of 50, particularly if right ventricular disease or established atrial fibrillation are present, the benefits of closure are even less easy to demonstrate and operative risk is higher. Nevertheless, two series involving patients over 60 to 65 years of age have demonstrated marked improvement in symptoms after surgical closure and shown that closure is feasible with acceptable risk in this population. However, no controlled clinical trial of closure will ever be performed with long-term follow-up, and cardiologists will continue to base the decision for closure in the older patient upon anecdotal evidence and uncontrolled series. Long-term results of those operated upon in the first two decades are excellent, although late atrial arrhythmias some 20 years post surgery still develop. Results of those operated upon in the third and fourth decades are still good but survival is less than that of an age-matched group. Repair after the age of 40 is associated with a significantly reduced late survival compared to age-matched controls because of cerebral vascular complications and atrial arrhythmias.

Ostium primum defect

Closure of the defect and repair of the mitral valve is indicated unless advanced pulmonary vascular disease is present. If the left atrioventricular valve anatomy is particularly abnormal, then repair may not be feasible and the combined procedure of repair of the ostium primum defect and mitral valve replacement should be considered. It may be advisable to delay this procedure if the patient is asymptomatic. Long-term follow up of patients following repair of the primum defect is good if pulmonary vascular disease and left atrioventricular valve regurgitation are absent. Late morbidity is related to atrial arrhythmias, atrioventricular block and progressive left atrioventricular valve regurgitation. They are all important and all of these patients require postoperative follow-up.

Summary

Most adult cardiologists will now see patients in whom atrial septal defects have been closed, and management will be directed to controlling arrhythmias and concomitant right ventricular disease or ischaemic and hypertensive left ventricular disease. If the defect is diagnosed for the first time in young adult life, then if a significant shunt is present and uncomplicated by pulmonary hypertension, it should be closed by surgery or transcatheter techniques if suitable. The decision in older patients with right ventricular disease and moderate elevation of pulmonary pressures is more difficult. The data from uncontrolled studies suggest that closure should still be considered, but over 50% of those undergoing repair in the fifth decade have persistent or new atrial dysrhythmias postoperatively. Heart–lung transplantation remains the only viable option for those with Eisenmenger syndrome.

Key references

Campbell M (1970) Natural history of atrial septal defect. *Br Heart J* **32**: 820–26.

Craig RJ, Selzer A (1968) Natural history and prognosis of atrial septal defects. *Circulation* **37**: 805–15.

Murphy JG, Gersh BJ, McGoon MD et al (1990) Long-term outcome after surgical repair of isolated atrial septal defect. Follow-up at 27 to 32 years. *N Engl J Med* **323**: 1645–50.

Nasrallah AT, Hall RJ, Garcia E, Leachman RD, Cooley, DA (1976) Surgical repair of atrial septal defect in patients over 60 years of age: Long-term results. *Circulation* **53**: 329–31.

Perloff JK (1984) Ostium secundum atrial septal defect – survival for 87 and 94 years. *Am J Cardiol* **53**: 388–89.

St John Sutton MG, Tajik AJ, McGoon DC (1981) Atrial septal defect in patients aged 60 years or older: Operative results and long-term postoperative follow-up *Circulation* **64**: 402–09.

12 Ventricular Septal Defect

In collaboration with Dr SJD Brecker

Introduction

Ventricular septal defect is the commonest congenital cardiac malformation in infants and children, but spontaneous or surgical closure make it less common in adults. Most adult patients with ventricular septal defects will fall into one of four groups: (i) those with previous surgical closure and no shunt; (ii) those with a small ventricular septal defect with a small shunt (<2:1) and normal right ventricular pressure (including those with a small residual defect post surgical closure); (iii) those with a moderate shunt and slight elevation of right ventricular pressure; and (iv) those with a large shunt with the Eisenmenger syndrome of severe pulmonary vascular disease and shunt reversal. Some patients with a large ventricular septal defect may be seen without the Eisenmenger syndrome if the pulmonary circulation has been protected by pulmonary valve or infundibular stenosis.

Key anatomical features

The anatomy of the interventricular septum is complex, and confusion may arise about the location of defects in this three dimensional structure. Defects may be classified into one of three morphological types defined on the basis of the structure forming the rim of the defect: perimembranous defects extend to involve the membranous septum (65% of total), muscular defects (30% of total) with entirely muscular rims which may be single or multiple, and doubly committed and subarterial defects (5%). Perimembranous and muscular defects may be further classified into inlet, trabecular and outlet defects depending upon the part of the interventricular septum involved. Thus a perimembranous inlet defect extends posteriorly to involve the inlet septum whereas a perimembranous outlet defect extends anteriorly beneath the semilunar valves (with malalignment of the outlet septum). Doubly committed subarterial defects are roofed by the fibrous continuity of the aortic and pulmonary valves and may be perimem-branous or muscular. They are usually unable to close spontaneously as the aortic valve forms the cephalad border, although with time an aortic cusp may prolapse into the defect and eventually seal it. When one of the aortic cusps (often the right coronary cusp) prolapses into a defect secondary aortic regurgitation may be present.

Pathophysiology

The physiology of all ventricular septal defects is that of a left to right shunt. It is dependent upon the size of the defect and shunt and the reaction of the pulmonary vasculature to the increased flow and hence relative resistances of the pulmonary and systemic circulations. Small defects offer high resistance to flow and a significant pressure drop may be generated across the defect (so called 'restrictive' ventricular septal defects). Pulmonary artery pressure will remain normal and the major risks of the adult with this defect are those of infective endocarditis. With a moderate-sized defect and shunt there may still be a significant pressure drop between the two ventricles, but pulmonary artery pressure will become mildly to moderately elevated. Serious pulmonary vascular disease and the Eisenmenger syndrome is unlikely unless the defect is large when almost no resistance to flow exists. In such situations the pulmonary circulation is exposed to systemic pressures. When pressures in the two ventricles are similar there may be little in the way of a murmur due to the defect but the signs of pulmonary hypertension will be impressive. If the pulmonary circulation is protected by pulmonary valvar or infundibular stenosis the physiology will be similar to that of Fallot's tetralogy (see Chapter 7).

Clinical findings

Symptoms

Small defects are usually asymptomatic and those with large enough shunts to be responsible for debilitating dyspnoea, exercise intolerance and respiratory infec-tions in childhood will be diagnosed and closed. Symptoms of infective endo-carditis are possible in all patients. Dyspnoea and exercise intolerance may develop secondary to worsening aortic regurgitation in those with defects close to the aortic valve, due to aortic cusp prolapse. Those with large non-restrictive defects will usually have the Eisenmenger syndrome by young adult life with cyanosis, markedly reduced exercise capacity, breathlessness, haemoptysis, angina, and palpitation secondary to atrial and ventricular arrhythmias.

Signs

The physical signs of a small ventricular septal defect in an adult are similar to those in childhood. The arterial and venous pulses are normal and there is a moderate or loud pansystolic murmur at the lower left sternal edge, but often audible towards the apex as well. There may be a systolic thrill at the left sternal edge. The pulmonary component of the second sound (P_2) is normal. Moderate-sized defects may lead to left ventricular volume overload with an active apex beat, and an early diastolic murmur of aortic regurgitation may be present in those defects associated with aortic cusp prolapse. In those adults with Eisenmenger syndrome, central cyanosis, clubbing, and the signs of pulmonary hypertension will be present: the venous pressure is raised with a dominant 'a' wave, the right ventricular impulse is prominent with a palpable P_2, and on auscultation there will be a right sided fourth sound, pulmonary ejection click and a loud P_2. Murmurs do not arise from the defect but from hypertension: thus an early diastolic murmur due to pulmonary regurgitation, a pansystolic murmur of tricuspid regurgitation.

Investigations

Electrocardiogram

The ECG of the patient with a small defect may be normal, but with a moderate sized defect there may be an increase in left ventricular voltages reflecting the volume loading. Left atrial and ventricular hypertrophy may be present in the adult with a moderate sized defect. The adult with Eisenmenger's syndrome will have right atrial and right ventricular hypertrophy. Postoperatively following closure the ECG will commonly show right bundle branch block.

Chest X-ray

This is normal in an adult with a small defect, but those with larger defects will show increased pulmonary vascular markings and increase in the size of the pulmonary arteries, the left atrium and the left ventricle. In the Eisenmenger syndrome, peripheral pruning of the pulmonary vasculature occurs.

Electrocardiography and Doppler

Two-dimensional echocardiography with colour flow Doppler usually identifies the type of defect clearly, although small defects less than 2 mm in width may be missed. The jet should however be detectable on continuous-wave Doppler even

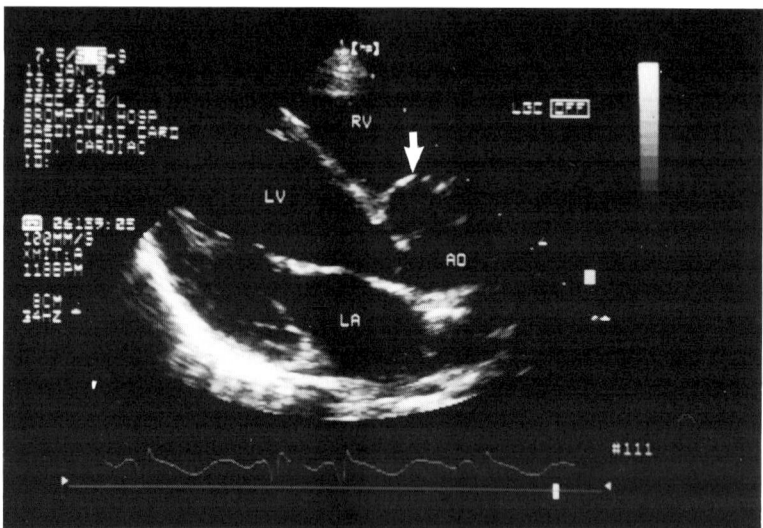

Figure 1. A small muscular outlet defect but with prolapse of the right coronary cusp of the aortic valve. Worsening aortic regurgitation can result and surgery is advisable if progression is demonstrable during follow-up.

from those defects not imaged. Perimembranous defects are identified by the characteristic echo dropout in the septum just adjacent to the central fibrous body and septal leaflet of the tricuspid valve. Muscular defects should be looked for throughout the length of the muscular septum and may be multiple. Subarterial defects are best demonstrated in the parasternal views, and aortic cusp prolapse may be clearly seen (Figure 1). In the Eisenmenger syndrome, the effects of pulmonary hypertension with right ventricular hypertrophy and septal displacement will be evident. Continuous-wave Doppler is used to calculate the pressure drop between the left and right ventricle. Knowing the systemic arterial blood pressure in the absence of aortic stenosis permits estimation of the peak right ventricular pressure by subtracting the LV–RV pressure drop from the blood pressure. Similarly, the peak tricuspid regurgitant velocity can be used to estimate pulmonary artery pressure if pulmonary stenosis is not present. Pulsed Doppler measurement of aortic and pulmonary artery flow can be used to estimate the pulmonary to systemic flow ratio.

Cardiac catheterization and angiography

Modern echocardiography and Doppler has made invasive investigation of these defects unnecessary for diagnosis. Saturation data can be used to calculate the magnitude of the shunt. The pulmonary vascular resistance may need to be determined if required when assessing patients for surgical closure or heart–lung transplantation.

Natural history

The natural history of a ventricular septal defect depends both upon its size and location, the relative pulmonary and systemic vascular resistances, and the effects of associated lesions. Almost half of all ventricular septal defects will close spontaneously. Indeed, 75% of defects not requiring early surgery will have closed by the age of 10 years. As stated, adults with small defects are not at risk of developing pulmonary vascular disease, but the risks of endocarditis are significant. Four per cent of all ventricular septal defect patients will develop endocarditis at some time in their lives, usually by the age of 40. The infection commonly occurs on the 'jet' lesion, the endocardial area traumatized by the high velocity blood impinging upon it through the defect. Aortic regurgitation is an important complication in some types of defect, and may be progressive. If such patients are not operated upon as children, worsening aortic regurgitation may lead to left ventricular disease, and surgery is required to halt this. Progressive pulmonary vascular disease is the most important complication of ventricular septal defects, and usually develops in the late teens or early twenties. Once this has occurred prognosis is poor, although survival to the fourth decade is possible. Heart–lung transplantation remains the only hope for such patients. In a small proportion of patients, right ventricular outflow tract obstruction may develop over the course of many years (sometimes known as two-chambered right ventricle). This is a rare cause of surgery in patients with small defects which would otherwise be left alone.

Pregnancy

Small defects should present no problems, but pregnancy should be avoided in those with severe pulmonary hypertension and the Eisenmenger syndrome. Those with moderate-sized defects and moderate pulmonary hypertension are at risk of developing left ventricular failure and rapidly worsening pulmonary hypertension during pregnancy.

Management of the adult with VSD

The asymptomatic patient with a small defect may be managed conservatively, but endocarditis prophylaxis is paramount. One episode of endocarditis how-ever has been used as strong grounds to close such a defect. Small to moderate-sized defects without symptoms may be followed closely, but many would advocate closure. Development of interventional techniques with trans-catheter devices may obviate the need for surgery in such cases. Occasionally an adult will be seen with a moderate to large defect and shunt but normal pulmonary artery pressures. These patients should probably undergo surgical closure to prevent further complications. Defects associated with aortic cusp prolapse and aortic regurgitation are likely to require surgical repair, and close follow-up with regard to timing of surgery is important. Asymptomatic patients with only mild aortic regurgitation may be followed, but early surgery is indicated if there is any indication of the regurgitation becoming more than mild. The development of pulmonary infundibular stenosis in a patient with a ventricular septal defect will adopt Fallot physiology and should be managed as such (see Chapter 7).

Patients with Eisenmenger syndrome represent the greatest challenge to the adult cardiologist. Death by the age of 40 years is the rule, and haemoptysis is a worrying symptom signifying pulmonary haemorrhage, infarction or not uncommonly thrombosis in situ. Polycythaemia is associated with hypoxia, dyspnoea, fatigue and thrombotic tendency, and regular venesections may be required. Simultaneous fluid replacement of colloid is important when venesecting such patients who tolerate hypotension extremely poorly. The possibility of cerebral abscess should be considered in any Eisenmenger patient with an alteration in mental state or focal neurological deficit. Travel to high altitudes is poorly tolerated and oxygen should be available if air travel is unavoidable. The greatest number of VSD patients that an adult cardiologist is likely to see will be those who have undergone surgical closure in childhood. Survival of these patients is good but not normal, and a number of late postoperative complications are recognized. These include atrioventricular block, ventricular arrhythmias, left ventricular disease, mitral tricuspid and aortic regurgitation, and progressive pulmonary vascular disease. The risk of infective endocarditis following closure is small as long as no residual defect remains, however prophylaxis is still recommended if there is any suggestion of a residual defect or valvular abnormalities are present.

Summary

Adult cardiologists will most commonly be faced with the patient who has undergone prior closure, or one with a large defect and the Eisenmenger syndrome. Management of the latter is not straightforward and should be undertaken by physicians seeing such patients frequently. New referrals may fall into one of two other categories – those who are asymptomatic with small defects who may be managed conservatively, and those with moderate defects in whom transcatheter closure or surgical repair should be considered. The importance of endocarditis prophylaxis cannot be overstated.

Key references

Campbell M (1971) Natural history of ventricular septal defect. *Br Heart J* **33**: 246–57.

Corone P, Doyon F, Gaudeau S et al (1977) Natural history of ventricular septal defect: A study involving 790 cases. *Circulation* **55**: 908–15.

Ellis JH IV, Moodie DS, Sterba R, Gill CC (1987) Ventricular septal defect in the adult: Natural and unnatural history. *Am Heart J* **114**: 115–20.

Otterstad JE, Nitter-Hauge S, Myhre E (1983) Isolated ventricular septal defect in adults: Clinical and haemodynamic findings. *Br Heart J* **50** 343–48.

Weidman WH, DuShane JW, Ellison RC (1977) Clinical course in adults with ventricular septal defect. *Circulation* **56**: I 78–I 79.

13 Coarctation of the Aorta

Introduction

Coarctation of the aorta may be associated with complex intracardiac abnormalities and is often the presenting problem whenever the aortic outflow tract is compromised. However, in this chapter we will concentrate on 'isolated' coarctation of the aorta with normal intracardiac connections.

Key anatomic features

Coarctation of the aorta is the commonest abnormality of the aortic arch. Its morphology varies with age. In neonates a sling of ductal tissue appears to be the most important anatomical problem, reduction in luminal size being related to constriction of ductal tissue. In older children and adults there is a fixed obstruction, usually distal to the left subclavian artery. This takes the form of a fibrous ridge, infolding or web, reducing the luminal diameter. It is probably a progressive lesion, and acquired atresia of the aortic arch at the site of a previous coarctation has been described. Lower body blood flow is maintained by the development of arterial collaterals which provide the basis for some of the clinical features of coarctation presenting in older life. The vessel wall proximal and distal to the coarctation segment may also be abnormal, with evidence of cystic medial necrosis. The intracardiac anatomy is variable. Bicuspid aortic valve is common and a VSD or history of VSD is a frequent association. Haemodynamically important mitral stenosis may be occult when there is severe coarctation and abnormalities of the left ventricular outflow tract (e.g. subaortic ridge) should be excluded in all patients with coarctation of the aorta.

Clinical features

Coarctation of the aorta in adults often presents with asymptomatic systemic hypertension. The reason for treating coarctation so aggressively in early life is because of the potential development of early cerebrovascular and coronary vascular disease and just occasionally patients with early myocardial infarction or cerebrovascular accident will have a peviously undiagnosed coarctation of the aorta. Palpation of the femoral pulses should be as routine a part of the examination of the adult cardiovascular system as it is in children. None the less, pulsatile femoral arteries may well be present in the presence of even severe coarctation of the aorta. This is due to the development of a collateral arterial supply to the lower body. The pulse pressure in the femoral arteries will almost always be reduced however, and radiofemoral delay under these circumstances will be marked. There will also be obvious continuous murmurs heard over the back particularly over both scapulae due to turbulent flow through the collaterals. Collateral flow tends to be less well developed when there is postoperative recoarctation. With the increasing trend towards performing subclavian flap angioplasty, it is worth remembering that a markedly diminished or inpalpable left brachial pulse is the norm, and that blood pressure measurements in the left arm may be misleading!

Further investigations

The chest radiograph may be normal but usually shows cardiomegaly. Over the age of 10 years there may be rib notching due to enlarged intercostal collateral arteries, but this is variable. Similarly, the electrocardiogram will vary from being entirely normal to showing gross left ventricular hypertrophy. Going along with this, cross-sectional echocardiography sometimes shows entirely normal left ventricular wall thickness even in the presence of severe coarctation. Indeed, the intracardiac anatomy may be entirely normal. Bicuspid aortic valve is more commonly seen however, and subtle abnormalities of the mitral valve apparatus will often be present if looked for. Direct visualization of the coarctation segment with cross-sectional imaging is difficult but the continuous wave Doppler examination from the suprasternal notch will show a characteristic descending aortic flow velocity spectral. There is an early high peak, but most importantly a long diastolic tail due to a continued gradient between ascending and descending aorta throughout the cardiac cycle (Figure 1).

Magnetic resonance imaging is the modality of choice for any abnormalities of the aortic arch (see Chapter 5). It is particularly useful in the follow-up of patients after surgery or catheter intervention, and is the only satisfactory way (short of angiography) of directly imaging the aortic arch under these circumstances.

Treatment

Because of the markedly increased risk of early cardiovascular and cerebro-vascular events, coarctation of the aorta should be adequately treated no matter

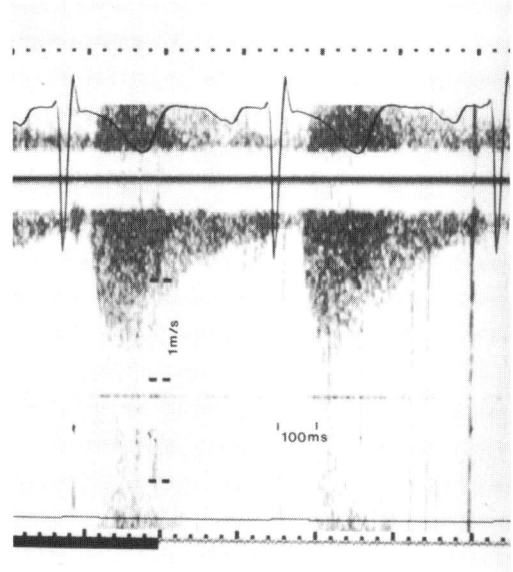

Figure 1. Continuous wave Doppler recording from the descending aorta of an adult with severe coarctation of the aorta. Although the peak gradient is low (10–15 mmHg) there is very characteristic diastolic 'tailing' to the spectral, reflecting a continued gradient throughout the cardiac cycle. The peak systolic gradient is low because of a very well-developed collateral circulation to the lower body.

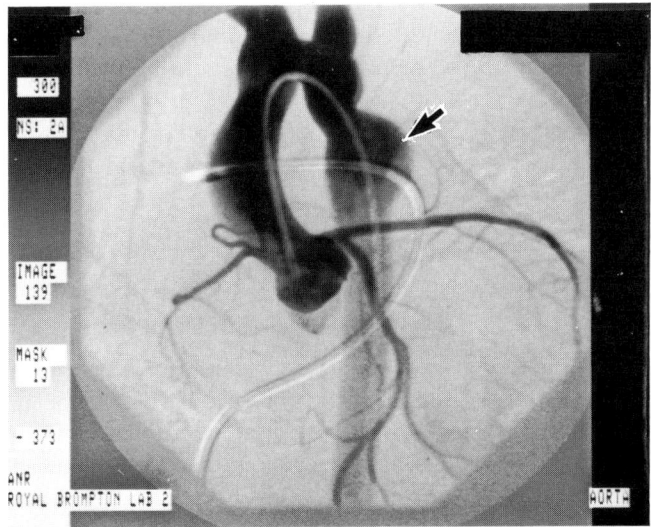

Figure 2. Subtracted aortogram showing an aortic aneurysm at the site of previous patch aortoplasty. This procedure has largely been abandoned.

what the age at presentation. Patch aortoplasty has now been largely abandoned because of the risk of subsequent aneurysm formation (Figure 2). However, surgical resection with end-to-end anastomosis is a very successful operation with a low mortality and very low risk of recoarctation when performed in adults. The alternative is balloon dilatation. This has the advantages of avoiding a thoracotomy and is successful in the majority of adults in whom it is attempted. There is a small risk of recoarctation, after a successful dilatation however (approx 10–20%) but, the most important long-term concern is that of aneurysm formation (see Chapter 19). Balloon dilatation of the aorta inevitably leads to dissection of the aortic wall. As mentioned above, the aortic wall around the site of coarctation may already be undermined and aneurysms of the aorta are seen in approximately 5–10% of cases. No deaths due to reported rupture of these aneurysms have yet been reported but this must be a particular risk, for example, in women of child-bearing age due to the additional hormonal effects of pregnancy further weakening the aortic wall. The technique has its protagonists but the majority of units have now moved away from this form of therapy for the treatment of coarctation of the aorta.

Recoarctation of the aorta

This is a more common problem in adults than primary coarctation of the aorta. There are two major approaches to surgical repair of coarctation in children, the end-to-end anastomosis, and subclavian flap repair. Both approaches have their supporters, and in good hands both procedures have acceptable results. It is probable, because of the circumferential anastomosis, that end-to-end anastomosis carries a higher long-term risk of recoarctation but this can occur with either procedure.

All patients previously operated upon for coarctation of the aorta require yearly or biannual review with assessment of their resting and exercise blood pressure and evidence of restenosis.

Management of recoarctation

Unlike native coarctation of the aorta the widely accepted treatment of first choice for recoarctation is balloon dilatation aortoplasty. Re-operation in these patients is hazardous, there being a risk of spinal cord damage due to interruption of spinal arterial flow, and this makes balloon dilatation more attractive. It is completely successful in three-quarters of patients (Figure 3) although in some the segment remains undilatable despite high pressure balloons. There is a small risk of aneurysm formation in this group but this complication seems more acceptable in view of the alternative surgical risks.

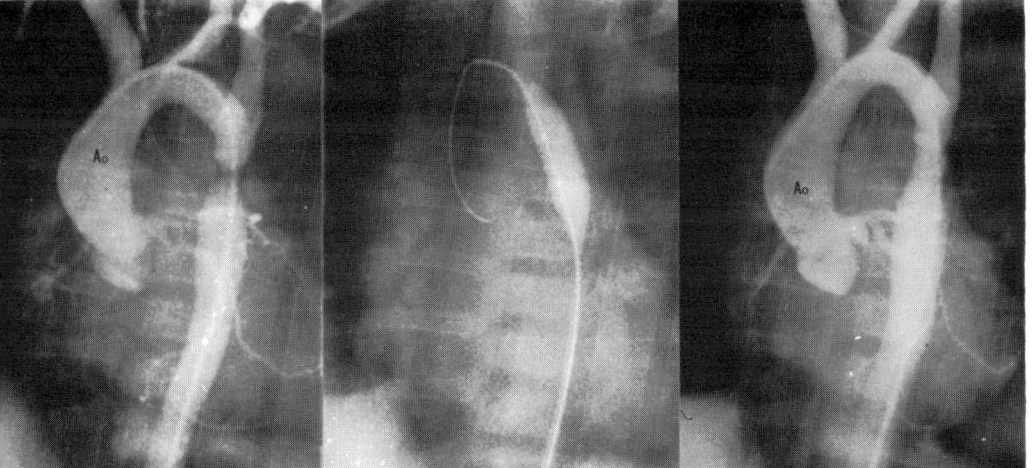

Figure 3. Balloon dilatation of recoarctation of the aorta. The restenosis is completely relieved following a single balloon inflation.

The surgical considerations are discussed in chapter 20 but suffice to say that if it is contemplated, then maintenance of lower body perfusion during surgery is mandatory.

Key references

Connor TM, Baker WP (1981) A comparison of coarctation resection and patch angioplasty using post exercise blood pressure measurements. *Circulation* **64**: 567–72.

Fawzy ME, Dunn B, Galal O et al (1992) Balloon coarctation angioplasty in adolescents and adults. Early and intermediate results. *Am Heart J* **123**: 674–80.

Hamilton D, Sandrasagra FA, Donnelly RJ (1978) Early and late results of aortoplasty with a left subclavian flap for coarctation of the aorta in infancy. *J Thorac Cadiovasc Surg* **75**: 699–704.

Presbitero P, Demarie D, Villani M et al (1987) Long-term results (15–30 years) of surgical repair of aortic coarctation. *Br Heart J* **57**: 462–67.

Wren C, Peart I, Bain H, Hunter S (1987) Balloon dilatation of unoperated aortic coarctation: Immediate results and 1 year follow-up. *Br Heart J* **58**: 369–73.

14 Aortic Valve Stenosis

In collaboration with Dr D Holdright

Introduction

Aortic stenosis is one of the most common congenital cardiac defects, account-ing for approximately 5% of all congenital heart disease presenting in infancy and childhood. Other forms of left ventricular outflow tract obstruction, for example supravalvar and subvalvar aortic stenosis, are recognized, but are less common and this chapter will confine itself to valvar lesions. In general, treatment of aortic stenosis in childhood is palliative, and ultimately valve replacement will be required in most. Later presentation implies milder disease but again the manage-ment of these patients should be pursued as if valve replacement is the likely endpoint.

Key anatomical features

In most instances in childhood the aortic valve is bicuspid, due to fusion of a commissure. Consequently, the orifice is eccentric and blood flow across the valve becomes turbulent. Rarely the valve is unicuspid and dome-shaped. In adults a tricuspid aortic valve may stenose, possibly triggered by minor irregu-larities and inequalities of the individual cusps. The congenitally bicuspid aortic valve thickens and becomes more rigid with time. About 10% have clinically detectable regurgitation which may not be apparent in the first few years of life. Calcium deposition within the valve is uncommon in childhood but occurs in adults, increasing with age, and is the most important long-term factor producing deterioration in later years. Normally functioning bicuspid valves and valves which are purely regurgitant rarely calcify in the first five decades. The precise trigger for calcium deposition is uncertain, but probably occurs as a result of wear and tear and the development of microthrombi which organize and subsequently calcify, creating a vicious spiral leading to further deterioration of the valve.

In isolated valvar aortic stenosis the aortic root may itself be small and the ascending aorta dilated. Aortic stenosis increases myocardial afterload, resulting in progressive and concentric left ventricular hypertrophy. Ultimately the left ventricle will dilate, this being an ominous feature reflecting end-stage disease.

Natural history

The natural history of unoperated aortic stenosis depends upon the severity of outflow tract obstruction, the speed with which it develops and the presence of associated cardiac malformations. Unoperated, the average life expectancy after the onset of symptoms is 5 to 10 yers, even less if heart failure is present. The stenotic valve frequently becomes regurgitant, the severity of which may alter the symptoms, signs and management of the patient.

Aortic stenosis is commonly classified as mild, moderate or severe. In the presence of preserved left ventricular function the pressure gradient across the aortic valve is a reasonable indicator of the severity of valve stenosis. Typically, a Doppler gradient of less than 40 mmHg is considered mild stenosis, between 40 and 70 mmHg is moderate stenosis and severe when higher. However, there are exceptions to the rule and the severity of the lesion should not be based solely on the pressure gradient measured across the valve.

Aortic stenosis may present in several different ways. In asymptomatic children and adolescents a heart murmur is often detected during routine examination. As aortic stenosis progesses there may be exertional chest pain and breathlessness. Typically, the pain is anginal in nature and usually occurs in the absence of atheromatous coronary artery disease. Subendocardial ischaemia results from a combination of left ventricular hypertrophy, increased wall tension and a raised left ventricular end-diastolic pressure. The use of vasodilators such as nitrates for chest pain should be avoided because they accentuate the haemodynamic effects of aortic stenosis. Dizziness, light-headedness and frank syncope generally reflect severe outflow tract obstruction and are indications for urgent surgery.

The aim in the remainder is correct timing of intervention. If left too late, left ventricular function may be irreversibly impaired. Conversely, premature intervention in the adolescent or young adult is equally undesirable since further operative procedures will inevitably be required in later life. In the unoperated state the degree of stenosis characteristically progresses over time, carrying with it the risk of sudden death. Since many cases of sudden death in patients with aortic stenosis are associated with physical activity and exertion, patients with moderate to severe aortic stenosis should avoid competitive sports and related activities. Although most cases of sudden death occur in patients with pre-existing symptoms, for example exertional breathlessness, chest pain and syncope, and in patients with ECG changes of left ventricular hypertrophy and strain pattern, the asymptomatic patient is not immune.

Progressive aortic stenosis results in compensatory left ventricular hypertrophy. In severe unoperated aortic stenosis left ventricular function ultimately declines, which has two main consequences. Not only may the classical signs of valve obstruction diminish or even disappear, making diagnosis at the bedside more difficult, but also perioperative mortality rises and the prognosis of survivors of aortic valve surgery diminishes.

In common with many congenital heart defects, aortic stenosis carries the risk of infective endocarditis, a risk which remains even in the operated state. Since there is no relationship between the severity of aortic stenosis and the risk of developing endocarditis all patients should be advised and treated similarly.

Palliation

Provided aortic regurgitation is not a dominant feature, aortic valvotomy, either surgical or by balloon valvuloplasty, may be undertaken. Surgical relief of aortic stenosis is performed under direct vision, after institution of cardiopulmonary bypass, by incision of the fused commissures. The procedure, which has been used for more than 30 years, is effective and carries a low perioperative mortality. Specific complications of surgical valvotomy include aortic regurgitation, residual obstruction and the possibility of restenosis. The presence of aortic regurgitation in the immediate postoperative period should be documented in order that the physical signs detected during follow-up may be interpreted correctly. The degree of aortic regurgitation may remain constant for many years whereas its development several years after valvotomy demands further investigation. Longitudinal studies indicate that the haemodynamic benefits of surgical valvotomy generally persist for many years. However, the operation must be considered palliative, especially in children, since one-third to one-half of patients will require reoperation within 10 years.

The use of balloon aortic valvuloplasty was first described in children in 1984 and in adults in 1986. Reduction of the stenosis is thought to result from commissural splitting. Performed percutaneously via the femoral artery the procedure is effective in children and young adults, but has largely been abandoned for senile calcific aortic stenosis. Complications include local vascular problems, arrythmias, aortic regurgitation and sudden death. The cited incidence of aortic regurgitation, which is the major complication following balloon valvuloplasty, varies from 15 to 33%. Regurgitation is usually mild but can be severe in some cases. In children the procedure generally achieves a reduction in gradient of up to 60%. Results are less good in young adults, probably because the valve is more heavily calcified and rigid. Paradoxically, residual aortic regurgitation is less of a problem and overall it is worth trying preoperative balloon dilatation in most patients with congenital aortic stenosis even if a previous surgical valvotomy is performed. Details are inappropriate, but

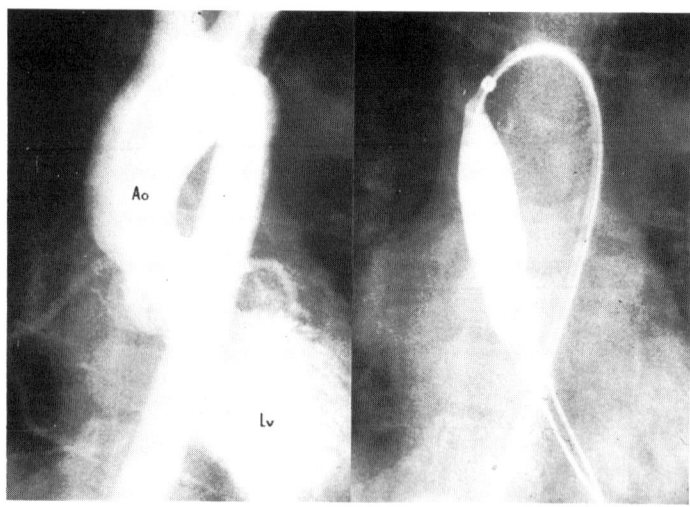

Figure 1. Balloon aortic valvotomy. It is important that the balloon size does not exceed the diameter of the aortic valve ring.

a balloon to aortic valve diameter ratio of greater than 0.9–1.0 should never be used (Figure 1).

Valve replacement

In those with failed palliation replacement with either a metal or bioprosthetic valve generally produces excellent symptomatic and haemodynamic relief. Surgical treatment in children and adolescents is less satisfactory since the implanted valve, whether metal or bioprosthetic, will not grow with the child. In addition, the lifespan of implanted valves is considerably less in this age group, and bioprosthetic valves are particularly prone to rapid degenerative change and calcification. Metal valves carry the added complication of long-term anticoagulant therapy, which is particularly difficult in active children. Consequently, valve replacement should be deferred as long as possible as should 'redo' valve surgery.

Many surgeons favour homograft aortic valve replacement should surgery be required before adulthood. Some centres use a pulmonary autograft, whereby the patient's own pulmonary valve is switched to the aortic position and a homograft is inserted in the pulmonary position. The rationale for this procedure is that the native pulmonary valve in the aortic position is more durable than the homograft aortic valve, that it may grow, and degeneration of the homograft valve is better tolerated in the pulmonary position. Long-term results are gradually becoming avoidable, but it is too early to say whether this is the surgical treatment of choice.

Clinical findings

Preoperative

The preoperative findings of aortic stenosis are similar in children and adults and need not be described in detail. However, an ejection click, preceding the ejection systolic murmur, is much more common in congenital aortic stenosis. As aortic stenosis progesses the click approaches the first heart sound, and becomes inaudible if the valve is heavily calcified and immobile. The aortic valve closure sound is also well preserved and occurs later in aortic stenosis such that the aortic component of the second heart sound may coincide with P_2 to produce a single second sound or may even occur after P_2, causing paradoxical splitting of the second heart sound.

Postoperative

The postoperative findings will of course depend on the extent to which the obstruction has been relieved. After successful valvotomy the character of the pulse and the pulse pressure return to normal. The left ventricular impulse becomes less forceful as left ventricular hypertrophy regresses. Similarly, the fourth heart sound usually disappears unless significant ventricular disease persists. A thrill should no longer be palpable. An ejection click usually remains audible. A soft ejection systolic murmur frequently persists after valvotomy and a new diastolic murmur may signify the development of postoperative aortic regurgitation.

After successful aortic valve replacement the physical signs similarly diminish. However, metal and bioprosthetic valves give rise to different auscultatory findings. Closure of metal valves, and sometimes opening, produces characteristic sounds. The systolic rumbling of a Starr-Edwards ball-and-cage valve in the aortic position should not be mistaken for persistent valve obstruction. There is considerable patient variability such that the 'ticking' noise of a normally functioning tilting-disc valve may be audible at the bedside in some patients whereas in others it can only be detected by auscultation. Occasionally a loud diastolic murmur is detectable postoperatively due to a small paravalvar leak of no haemodynamic significance. Such a murmur will persist during follow-up and does not require further investigation in its own right. A normally-functioning bioprosthetic aortic valve is indistinguishable by auscultation from a normal aortic valve.

Chest radiograph

Preoperative

The chest X-ray appearance may be unremarkable in aortic stenosis. With increasing stenosis left ventricular hypertrophy produces rounding of the cardiac apex. The cardiothoracic ratio is normal or slightly increased and post-stenotic dilatation of the aorta is frequently observed. Left atrial enlargement indicates severe aortic stenosis. Calcification within the aortic valve may be visible, particularly on the lateral chest X-ray.

Postoperative

Postoperatively the radiographic abnormalities resolve but some dilatation of the ascending aorta may persist. Late after bioprosthetic valve replacement calcification deposition may again be seen within the valve leaflets or, more commonly, the aortic wall supporting the leaflets.

Electrocardiogram

Preoperative

Sinus rhythm is usual but in severe cases P mitrale or atrial fibrillation may develop. The electrocardiogram frequently shows changes of left ventricular hypertrophy with strain pattern. With progressive stenosis deep S waves develop in leads V_1 and V_2 and the T waves in the lateral leads flatten and then invert. With time the degenerative calcific process can involve the conduction system to cause variable degrees of atrioventricular block, left axis deviation and left bundle branch block.

Postoperative

After corrective surgery the electrocardiographic changes of left ventricular hypertrophy improve, but frequently the ECG remains abnormal. Intraventricular conduction defects may persist and the development of preoperative left bundle branch block is usually permanent.

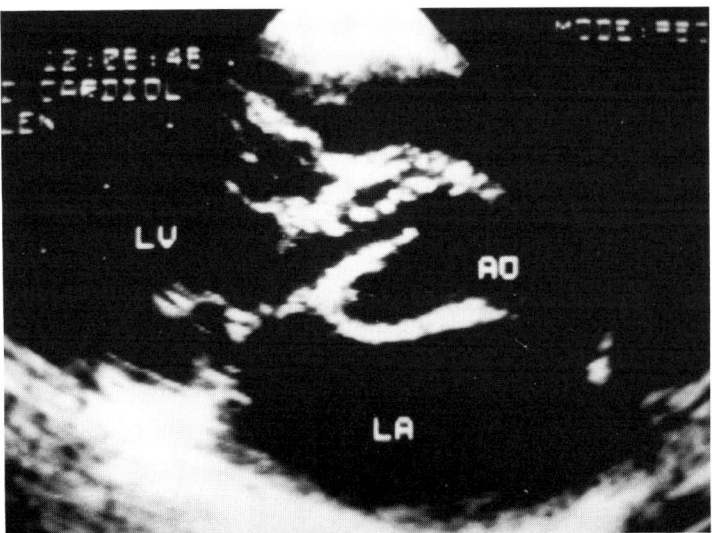

Figure 2.   Cross-sectional echocardiogram of a bicuspid aortic valve in long-axis projection. Note the thickened leaflets with a characteristically markedly eccentric opening.

Cross-sectional echocardiography and Doppler studies ———

Preoperative

Cross-sectional echocardiography demonstrates uniform hypertrophy of the left ventricle. The left atrium may be enlarged and minor abnormalities of the mitral valve are common. The aortic valve leaflets are thickened and may be calcified, with diminished systolic excursion easily demonstrated by M-mode echocardiography, which may also reveal eccentric valve opening and closure (Figure 2). Dilatation of the ascending aorta is readily detected. The right heart chambers are of normal size unless significant pulmonary hypertension exists. Doppler studies will demonstrate increased forward velocity across the aortic valve, but more than one window should be used to minimize the risk of underestimating the severity of the stenosis. Varying degrees of aortic regurgitation may also be found and functional mitral regurgitation into a dilated left atrium may be present.

Postoperative

Transthoracic echocardiography is more difficult in patients with previous cardiac surgery but usually the valve can be visualized in one of the standard views. Doppler velocities across metal valves in the aortic position are slightly higher than normal and vary according to the valve type. Whereas small regurgitant jets may be a normal finding in healthy subjects, any degree of regurgitation through or around a metal valve is abnormal. Metal valves create acoustic echoes which make cross-sectional imaging of neighbouring structures difficult, which is particularly important if infective endocarditis is suspected and the presence of an aortic root abscess or vegetations on the valve are being sought. In such instances transoesophageal studies may be useful.

Cardiac catheterization with angiography

In many patients cardiac catheterization adds little or nothing to the information which can be obtained with non-invasive methods. Thus, the aims of cardiac catheterization are to confirm or refute the diagnosis in patients who are poor echo subjects or where data from non-invasive tests are inconclusive, and to look for coexisting coronary artery disease in much older patients. Occasionally, additional abnormalities may be discovered at catheterization which previously had gone undetected, for example mild aortic coarctation. Left ventriculography and aortography add further information regarding the outflow tract and aortic root which might prove important at the time of surgery.

The gradient recorded during pull-back of the catheter across the aortic valve is usually less than that recorded by Doppler ultrasound, which measures the peak instantaneous gradient. If cardiac output is measured at cardiac catheterization the aortic valve area can be calculated, which is helpful if balloon valvuloplasty is to be performed. Crossing the stenotic valve with the catheter may be difficult from the femoral approach and is generally easier when performed via the brachial artery or in very small children, from the carotid. Sometimes the valve cannot be crossed retrogradely from the ascending aorta and a trans-septal puncture, entering the left ventricle from the right atrium through the atrial septum may be necessary. However, catheterization in these patients is not without risk and should only be undertaken if adequate information cannot be obtained by less invasive methods.

Specific postoperative problems

Thrombosis and embolism are problems of valve replacement, no matter what age the surgery is performed. Anticoagulation regimes are similar to those in acquired heart disease and need not be discussed further.

Complete heart block may develop after aortic valve replacement, particularly if there is extensive calcification present. This rhythm may be transient, lasting only a few days, or may be persistent and necessitate permanent pacing. In some patients this may be predicted at operation and an endocardial system can be implanted at the same time. Patients with transient perioperative complete heart block should be followed carefully for the development of conduction defects in later life.

Whatever form of palliative or corrective surgery the patient remains at risk of endocarditis throughout life. Endocarditis still carries a significant mortality, particularly if associated with a prosthetic valve. The infection may never be completely eradicated. Therefore scrupulous attention to dental hygiene and appropriate antibiotic prophylaxis for dental and surgical procedures are required.

Summary

Aortic stenosis remains a common congenital heart defect which, if unrecognized, carries a high mortality. Relief of the obstruction can be obtained in several ways with excellent results. Perhaps the most difficult aspect of managing young patients with aortic stenosis is knowing when to operate. The decision is relatively straightforward in mild and severe cases, but careful assessment is essential in those patients who appear to fall between these two extremes.

Key references

Kitchiner D, Jackson K, Walsh K, Peart I, Arnold R (1994) The progression of mild congenital aortic valve stenosis from childhood into adult life. *Int J Cardiol* **42** (3): 217–25.

Matsuki O, Robles A, Gibbs J et al (1988) Long-term performance of 555 aortic homografts in the aortic position. *Ann Thorac Surg* **46**: 187.

Sullivan ID, Wren C, Bain H et al (1989) Balloon dilatation of the aortic valve for congenital aortic stenosis in childhood. *Br Heart J* **61**: 186.

15 Pulmonary Valve Stenosis

In collaboration with Dr D Holdright

Introduction

Pulmonary valve stenosis is a common congenital heart defect, accounting for 7–8% of all cases. It may occur in isolation or as part of a more complex cardiac problem. Although the precise aetiology remains unknown, pulmonary stenosis may be associated with various genetic, chromosomal or environmental factors. Characteristically, pulmonary stenosis occurs more frequently in siblings rather than in successive generations. Pulmonary stenosis in association with skeletal and facial abnormalities reminiscent of Turner's syndrome, but in the presence of a normal karyotype, is known as Noonan's syndrome. Noonan's syndrome is inherited as an autosomal dominant condition with variable penetrance and the characteristic features of the condition may be seen to a greater or lesser extent in other family members.

Key anatomical features

The pulmonary valve is typically dysplastic. The poorly formed valve cusps are thickened and valve excursion is consequently limited. There is frequently an element of narrowing at the sinutubular junction, at the level of the superior attachment of the leaflets in the pulmonary artery. With increasing valve stenosis the right ventricle hypertrophies. Localized infundibular hypertrophy may, paradoxically, worsen the degree of obstruction. In severe cases the right ventricle dilates and the stretched tricuspid valve ring results in tricuspid regurgitation. Ultimately, progressive tricuspid regurgitation and right atrial hypertension leads to venous engorgement and right heart failure. At this stage right-to-left shunting may occur at atrial level through a stretched foramen ovale.

Natural history

Compared with aortic valve stenosis, stenosis of the pulmonary valve is generally better tolerated and is associated with a more benign course. In some children the severity of stenosis actually diminishes as the child grows. This is more common in patients with mild stenosis where the increase in valve orifice size is proportionally greater than the increase in cardiac output. In severe pulmonary stenosis in infancy the haemodynamic significance of the lesion increases with growth of the child. Severe pulmonary stenosis presenting in the neonate is frequently associated with a hypoplastic right ventricle and is fatal without intervention.

Older patients with isolated pulmonary stenosis generally do very well for many years. Indeed, severe pulmonary stenosis causing symptoms in childhood is uncommon. Typically a cardiac murmur is picked up at routine medical examination of an otherwise healthy child. Mild pulmonary stenosis, with a Doppler-derived pressure gradient of less than 40 mmHg across the valve, and moderate stenosis (less than 60 mmHg gradient) may be found in asymptomatic adults and are compatible with a near-normal lifespan. Symptoms may not be present even in severe pulmonary stenosis. When symptoms develop the patient typically describes fatigue and breathlessness due to low cardiac output on exercise. In severe cases chest pain and syncope develop, heralding the risk of sudden death unless intervention is performed.

Intervention

To consider intervention for pulmonary stenosis as being either palliative or corrective is somewhat artificial, since pulmonary valve replacement is rarely required in isolated pulmonary stenosis. The results of surgical valvotomy or balloon valvuloplasty are excellent in most cases, and the haemodynamic result is usually long-lasting.

Intervention is usually considered when the gradient across the pulmonary valve exceeds 50 to 60 mmHg. For many years open valvotomy was the treatment of choice, producing excellent haemodynamic results at very low risk. However, in the last ten years surgical valvotomy has been replaced by balloon valvuloplasty as the treatment of choice. The current technique of balloon valvuloplasty was first described in 1982 and, nowadays, it is the commonest interventional procedure performed at catheterization in children.

Balloon valvuloplasty of the pulmonary valve is effective and safe. It works by causing commissural splitting of the stenotic valve. Rarely there is evidence of cusp tearing and avulsion. Any secondary pulmonary regurgitation is usually well-tolerated and usually less severe than after surgery. The technique, which is relatively easy to perform, involves crossing the stenotic valve and inflation of

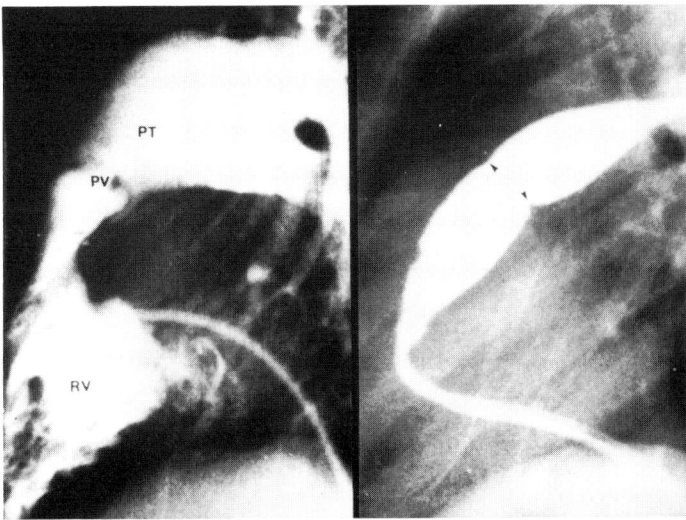

Figure 1.   Severe valvar pulmonary stenosis in an adult. Note the doming valve, infundibular systolic narrowing and poststenotic dilatation of the pulmonary artery. A single 25 mm balloon has been used (right-hand panel) and the valve 'waist' is virtually abolished (arrowed).

a balloon matched in size to the valve annulus. Subsequent inflations with a slightly oversized balloon generally produce a better gradient reduction with a lower incidence of restenosis (Figure 1). In adolescents and adults a double balloon technique may be needed.

When the valve is very dysplastic neither surgical valvotomy nor valvuloplasty is the surgical treatment of choice since the obstruction is not due to commissural fusion. In such instances excision of the valve leaflet(s) with or without patch enlargement or valve replacement is required. Sometimes the right ventricular outflow itself must be enlarged by insertion of a patch, together with resection of the hypertrophied subvalvar myocardium.

Clinical findings

Preoperative

With increasing pulmonary stenosis the signs of right heart failure may be detected. Cyanosis may be both peripheral, due to a low output state, or central, due to right-to-left shunting at atrial level. The jugular venous pulse is characteristically abnormal. Giant 'a' waves, which coincide with a right-ventricular fourth heart sound, are due to a non-compliant right ventricle. These physical signs are lost if atrial fibrillation develops. The precordial impulse may be abnormal due to right ventricular hypertrophy.

The second heart sound is widely split, with a diminished pulmonary component. The delay in P_2 increases with increasingly severe stenosis. An ejection click, produced by doming of the valve at its point of maximum excursion, may be heard in the pulmonary area if the valve is mobile but is absent if the valve is dysplastic. The ejection systolic murmur is typically loud and long, and is easily heard in the pulmonary area and transmitted to the neck. As the severity of pulmonary stenosis increases, the duration of the systolic murmur also increases due to a prolonged right ventricular ejection time. In mild stenosis the murmur, which is characteristically soft and symmetrical in shape, ends before the aortic component (A_2) of the second heart sound. As the stenosis increases in severity, so the murmur extends beyond A_2, which is obliterated in severe pulmonary stenosis.

Postoperative

The jugular venous waveform returns toward normal, although a prominent 'a' wave may be seen in the presence of persistent right ventricular dysfunction, which is more likely in older patients. In the absence of residual obstruction the second heart sound splits normally. The systolic murmur diminishes in intensity and duration and an immediate diastolic murmur due to pulmonary regurgitation may be present.

Chest radiograph

Preoperative

The chest X-ray may be normal in mild pulmonary stenosis. The heart size is frequently normal, and only enlarges in severe cases where dilatation of the right ventricle occurs. An enlarged right atrium may be seen. The most striking abnormality is poststenotic dilatation of the main pulmonary artery. The left pulmonary artery is also enlarged, due to the high velocity jet across the stenotic valve which is directed preferentially into the left pulmonary artery. The degree of pulmonary artery dilatation is unrelated to the severity of the stenosis. Calcification of the pulmonary valve may be seen in adults.

Postoperative

Characteristically the pulmonary artery remains dilated, even after successful relief of the stenosis. The heart size returns towards normal and the right ventricle and right atrium are no longer prominent. With time, calcification may develop in the pulmonary valve.

Electrocardiogram

Preoperative

In mild cases the ECG is normal. With increasing pulmonary stenosis the right ventricle hypertrophies, to produce characteristic ECG changes. The QRS axis in the frontal plane deviates to the right. Right bundle branch block, partial or complete, may be present. The R wave amplitude in leads V_4R and V_1 increases such that the R wave amplitude exceeds that of the ensuing S wave. Deep S waves develop in the lateral precordial leads. The T waves in leads V_4R and V_1 are initially peaked but subsequently invert. With worsening pulmonary stenosis right atrial enlargement produces P pulmonale.

Postoperative

The ECG becomes less abnormal postoperatively as right ventricular hypertrophy regresses. The tall R waves in leads V_4R and V_1 diminish and the T waves normalize.

Cross-sectional echocardiography and Doppler studies

Preoperative

The pulmonary artery and pulmonary valve are best visualized in the parasternal short axis and subcostal views. The most characteristic finding is doming of the pulmonary valve in systole. Presystolic opening of the valve, due to an elevated right ventricular end-diastolic pressure in severe pulmonary stenosis, can be recognized on M-mode examination. The dilated pulmonary artery is readily visualized on 2D echocardiography and because of the location of the pulmonary valve the severity of the stenosis can be accurately determined by Doppler echocardiography using the short axis parasternal approach.

Postoperative

Echocardiography is a useful method for following patients postoperatively to look for evidence of restenosis. Following valvotomy or valvuloplasty varying degrees of pulmonary regurgitation may be found, which is usually well-tolerated.

Cardiac catheterization with angiography

Cardiac catheterization should only be necessary if pulmonary valvuloplasty is contemplated. The stenotic pulmonary valve can be difficult to cross since the orifice is often extremely small. A right coronary catheter is often perfectly shaped to direct a wire through the valve in these circumstances. Obstruction to forward flow of blood across the valve by the catheter occasionally produces haemodynamic collapse, which is rapid in onset. If balloon valvuloplasty is to be performed the end-hold catheter is positioned in a distal pulmonary artery and then exchanged over a wire for a balloon dilatation catheter. When the balloon is straddling the pulmonary valve, it is inflated until the waist disappears (Figure 1). If very severe an intravenous dose of 0.1 mg/kg of propranolol should be given intravenously during balloon deflation, and repeated if severe muscular dynamic obstruction persists after relief of the valve gradient.

Specific postoperative problems

Pulmonary regurgitation may develop after balloon valvuloplasty. It is usually mild and is well tolerated. Severe regurgitation is rare. Arrhythmias may occur at the time of valvuloplasty but are usually short-lived and resolve spontaneously.

Summary

Pulmonary stenosis is a common congenital heart defect which, in most cases, is well-tolerated and has a relatively benign course. Because of the success of balloon valvuloplasty in this condition, surgical valvotomy is no longer the treatment of choice in infants and adolescents. The results are less good in adults in whom surgery may still play a role.

Key references

Stanger P, Cassidy SC, Girod DA et al (1990) Balloon pulmonary valvuloplasty: Results of the valvuloplasty and angioplasty of congenital anomalies registry. *Am J Cardiol* **65**: 775.

16 Ebstein's Anomaly

In collaboration with Dr S Cullen

Introduction

The natural history of Ebstein's anomaly is extremely variable. It may present at any age, and is associated with a variety of haemodynamic and electrophysiological sequelae. The more severe the deformity of the tricuspid valve the earlier the presentation and even interuterine death is recognized. At the other end of the spectrum late presentation in adult life may occur when there is only mild abnormality of the tricuspid valve.

Key morphological features

Ebstein's anomaly may occur in isolation or can be associated with other congenital heart defects (see Chapter 17). The hallmark in this anomaly is apical displacement of thickened septal and/or mural leaflets of the tricuspid valve with atrialization of part of the right ventricle. In the normal heart the atrioventricular septum is defined by normal offsetting between the tricuspid and mitral valves. Normally the tricuspid valve is displaced with the apex of the right ventricle. The upper limit of normal of the distance between the septal attachments of the mitral and tricuspid valves is approximately 1.5 cm in a normal adult heart. The valve itself can be stenotic, normally functioning, or regurgitant.

Associated cardiac defects, apart from patent foramen ovale or atrial septal defect occur in approximately 30% of cases and are common in the younger age groups. Right ventricular outflow tract obstruction is particularly common ranging from mild valvar pulmonary stenosis to pulmonary atresia. Ebstein's anomaly of the left atrioventricular valve may occur in the setting of corrected transposition and in this setting additional aortic arch abnormalities may be present.

Presentation

The mode of presentation is age-dependent. There is an early death hazard due to haemodynamic sequelae of severe tricuspid valve displacement. Severe right ventricular hypoplasia leads to extreme cyanosis whereas severe tricuspid regurgitation may cause heart failure and death in the neonatal period. Inter-uterine cardiomegaly results in pulmonary hypoplasia when there is a high incidence of fetal loss with this abnormality. An incidental cardiac murmur may be the only finding in older children. Arrhythmia represents the major problem in adolescents and adults with Ebstein's anomaly. There is a well-recognized association with pre-excitation on the electrocardiogram (Wolfe Parkinson White syndrome) and the risk of tachyarrhythmias may be increased by progressive atrial dilation. The more severe the tricuspid valve regurgitation the greater the likelihood of right ventricular outflow tract obstruction resulting from low antegrade flow during development of the outflow tract.

Investigations

The cardiothoracic ratio on chest X-ray may be increased, reflecting the right atrial dilatation secondary to the tricuspid valve regurgitation. The typical finding on standard 12-lead electrocardiogram is prolonged PR interval, right atrial enlargement, superior axis with or without right bundle branch block pattern. Approximately, 20% of patients will have overt pre-excitation on the resting electrocardiogram (Wolfe Parkinson White syndrome).

The advent of cross-sectional echocardiography has greatly facilitated the diagnosis of Ebstein's anomaly. All of its features are readily recognized using subcostal and apical four-chamber use. The deformity of the tricuspid valve can be defined as can the extent of tricuspid valve regurgitation using colour Doppler echocardiography. Because of the high incidence of associated defects a detailed examination of the whole heart is required.

In the classical cases of Ebstein's anomaly there is no place for cardiac catheterization which in the past has been associated with serious morbidity and mortality. In patients with arrhythmias electrophysiological study is under-taken with a view to radiofrequency ablation of accessory pathways. The accessory connections may be single or multiple and are classically found in the right posteroseptal region.

Predictors of outcome

The earlier the presentation, the higher the risk of death. Thus presentation during fetal life is associated with a high mortality. A cardiothoracic ratio greater than 60%, severe right ventricular outflow tract abnormalities and the greater the dimension of the right atrium relative to the other chambers of the heart are all associated with an increased risk of death. Interestingly, the presence or absence of pre-excitation on the electrocardiogram does not appear to be a risk factor for mortality.

Surgical intervention

Tricuspid valve regurgitation may produce severe heart failure and/or associated cyanosis and usually prompts the question of surgical intervention. It is interesting to note that in most large series it is surgery itself which tends to be the biggest risk factor for death not withstanding the underlying haemodynamic abnormalities. In the neonate the indications for operation are usually persistent cyanosis with or without associated heart failure, whereas severe heart failure with or without arrhythmias are more common in the older subjects. Tricuspid valve surgery and replacement has been undertaken across the whole age spectrum. The older the patient the better the outlook with the highest preoperative mortality usually noted in the first year of life. In contrast with the adult presentation, the Ebstein's anomaly may be so severe in neonatal life or associated with other cardiac anomalies that conventional surgery has no place. In those cases cardiac transplantation or innovative surgical techniques leading to an eventual Fontan-type circulation have been undertaken.

Associated problems

Paradoxical embolus may rarely occur in the setting of Ebstein's anomaly. But routine anticoagulation is not necessary for all patients in sinus rhythm. The risk of endocarditis on the tricuspid valve is extremely low. Arrhythmias are common, especially in older patients and are frequently associated with accessory atrioventricular connections. Catheter ablation of the accessory pathways is now performed but is a more difficult procedure because of the position of the pathway. Atrial flutter and fibrillation are also common arrhythmias and may be resistant to drug treatment.

Left ventricular dysfunction is sometimes seen during long-term follow-up. Patchy fibrosis of the right and left ventricular myocardium, but clinical symptoms of left ventricular are rare.

Summary

Ebstein's anomaly may present at any age and the natural history is extremely variable. The clinical features, age of presentation, presence of associated defects and severity of the tricuspid valve regurgitation dictate the management. When it presents in fetal life the outlook is awful. During childhood with rare exceptions, medical management is the rule. If this fails, surgical repair or replacement of the tricuspid valve may have a place but only as a last resort. Arrhythmia such as atrial fibrillation and flutter become more common with increasing age and should be treated medically in the first instance.

Key references

Celermajer DS, Bull C, Till JA, et al (1994) Ebsteins Anomaly: Presentation and outcome from fetus to adult. *J Amer Coll Cardiol* **23**: 170–76.

Watson H (1974) Natural history of Ebstein's anomaly of tricuspid valve in childhood and adolescence: An international cooperative study of 505 cases. *Br Heart J* **36**: 417–27.

17 Corrected Transposition of the Great Arteries

In collaboration with Dr A Bishop

Introduction

When Rokitansky first described this condition, in 1875, he noted that in some cases of transposition of the great arteries the anomaly was 'corrected by the position of the ventricular septum'. By this he meant that although the aorta arose from the morphological right ventricle and the pulmonary artery from the morphological left ventricle, the blood from the right atrium (systemic venous return) entered the ventricle from which arose the pulmonary artery, and blood from the left atrium (pulmonary venous return) entered the ventricle giving rise to the aorta. The condition has since been called **corrected transposition**. Segmentally, congenitally corrected transposition consists of a discordant atrioventricular and ventriculo-arterial connection.

The clinical features of this syndrome were described by Anderson in 1957, and since then its natural history, associations, and surgical management have become well known. It represents approximately 0.5% of all diagnosed congenital heart defects, and is slightly more common in males. The majority of cases presenting in childhood have severe complicating abnormalities. The exact prevalance is, however, unknown. This is because corrected transposition without those association anomalies may remain undiagnosed and only be detected post mortem. None the less, complete heart block, left atrioventricular valve dysfunction and systemic ventricular failure may all lead to presentation in adult life.

Anatomy

The normal relationships of atria, ventricles, and great vessels, are the result of rotation of the embryonic bulboventricular loop, and it is not difficult to construct a theory of malrotation that explains the basic abnormality of corrected transposition. While the condition is most easily understood by assuming simple switching of right and left ventricles, the actual anatomical arrangement of the cardiac structures is more complex than this.

In the most common arrangement the atria are normally positioned with normal connections to vena cavae, and pulmonary veins (situs solitus). The atria connect to the ventricles through a mitral and tricuspid valve. The atrioventricular valves develop in continuity with the ventricles, so that the mitral valve allows blood from the right atrium into the right sided ventricle which has left ventricular morphology. The mitral valve is not a common site for clinically significant lesions, but in one series of post mortem examinations more than 50% of valves had an abnormality, with abnormal cusp number, or papillary muscles, cleft anterior leaflets and occasional congenital stenosis. The tricuspid valve connects the left atrium to the morphological right ventricle and is a common site for clinically important abnormalities. Approximately 30% of patients with corrected transposition will have significant tricuspid valve incompetence, but at post mortem more than 90% have tricuspid anomalies. The three cusps in this condition are anterior, inferior, and septal, and these are commonly dysplastic. In addition the septal and inferior cusps may be displaced apically; rarely there is a full Ebstein type anomaly, with atrialization of the ventricle proximal to the valve ring (Figure 1). A ventricular septal defect is particularly common in such cases.

The ventricles usually lie side-by-side in the chest with the left sided ventricle having right ventricular morphology. Thus, it is coarsely trabeculated, and has a

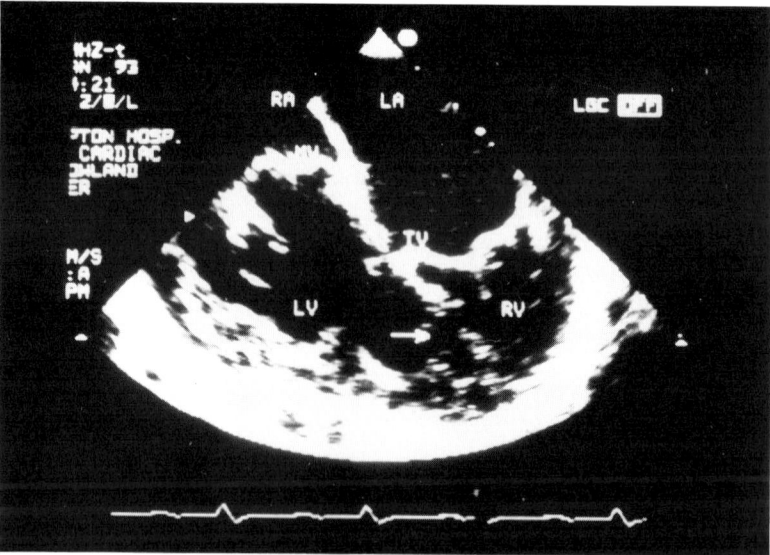

Figure 1. Transoesophageal echocardiogram. The right atrium (RA) is connected to the left ventricle (LV). The left atrium (LA) is markedly enlarged because of apical displacement of the septal leaflet of the tricuspid valve (TV) (Ebstein's anomaly of the tricuspid valve). There is also a ventricular septal defect (arrowed).

separate muscular infundibular chamber giving rise to the aorta. There is therefore no continuity between the left sided AV and VA valves. The position of the
infundibulum is such that the aorta arises anterior, and to the left of the
pulmonary artery. Conversely, there is usually fibrous continuity between the
mitral and pulmonary valve. The semilunar valve connecting the right sided
ventricle to the pulmonary artery is a pulmonary valve, and that between the
left sided ventricle and the aorta is an aortic valve, giving rise to left, right and
anterior aortic sinuses.

The left and right sinuses are usually posterior and give rise to left and right
coronary arteries. The coronary distribution reflects the ventricular inversion; the
left runs in the right atrioventricular groove. The right coronary artery runs in
front of the pulmonary outflow tract. Since pulmonary stenosis is a common
association, surgery in this area is common, and preservation of the right
coronary is part of the rationale for the increasing use of right ventricle to
pulmonary artery conduits in surgery for the relief of right sided ventricular
outflow tract obstruction.

The conducting tissues in corrected transposition are also abnormally distributed. In the normal heart the atrioventricular node lies at the base of the
atrioventricular canal at the origin of the membranous septum. In the heart
with corrected transposition the pulmonary artery and valve are positioned deep
between the mitral and tricuspid valve rings and the adjacent membranous
septum is often deficient, leaving a subpulmonary ventricular septal defect.
There is usually an anterior AV node and the bundle from this runs anterior
to the pulmonary outflow tract before branching. The main bundle is therefore
vulnerable to surgical disruption during repair of a VSD, or relief of pulmonary
outflow tract obstruction. This is the main reason for the increasing use of
bypassing conduits in the relief of pulmonary obstruction.

Associated lesions

If the clinically insignificant anomalies of the morphologically tricuspid (left
sided) valve are included, the incidence of associated lesions in corrected
transposition has been reported as high as 90%.

Ventricular septal defect

The incidence of VSD in correct transposition is approximately 80%. It is an
almost universal finding if there is significant apical displacement of the tricuspid
valve. The defect is usually in the membranous septum, beneath the pulmonary
valve. The defect is usually large, leading to a substantial left-to-right shunt
(unless there is coexisting pulmonary outflow obstruction) and pulmonary
vascular disease may therefore result.

Pulmonary outflow obstruction

Some degree of valvar or subvalvar pulmonary stenosis occurs in 60–70% of cases, and in 80% of those with a VSD. Subvalvar stenosis may be caused by a fibrous ring, an accumulation of fibrous or myxomatous tissue, or by the presence of a muscular tunnel in the outflow tract. While the presence of pulmonary stenosis may protect the pulmonary vessels from a left-to-right shunt through a VSD, the stenosis may ultimately result in a right-to-left shunt cyanosis. The balance between the VSD and the outflow tract obstruction, however, may be such that the patient survives without severe pulmonary vascular disease or cyanosis into adult life.

Left atrioventricular valve regurgitation

The almost universal anomalies of the morphological tricuspid valve in corrected transposition result in clinically significant incompetence in approximately 30% of cases. While those valves with full Ebstein type anatomy are grossly incompetent at birth, more commonly the systemic ventricular dilatation that occurs with time will exacerbate mild or moderate regurgitation, and cause gradual clinical deterioration. Tricuspid regurgitation is therefore a comparatively common cause of presentation in the adult or adolescent (Figure 2).

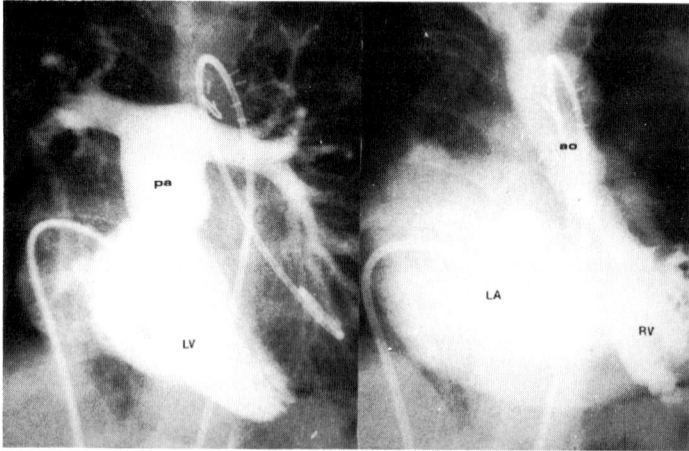

Figure 2. Anteroposterior projections of left (LV, left hand panel) and right (RV, right hand panel) ventriculograms. There is severe tricuspid (systemic atrioventricular) valve regurgitation with massive enlargement of the left atrium (LA).

Other associations

Table 1.   Associations described in corrected transposition with increased frequency, although remaining uncommon in this context

Atrial septal defect
Patent ductus arteriosus
Mitral valve dysplasia
Subvalvar aortic obstruction
Aortic arch hypoplasia
Coarctation of the aorta

Electrophysiological abnormalities

Because of the abnormal atrioventricular connections in this condition, defective conduction and pre-excitation are common. The presence of an anterior atrioventricular node and the abnormal anterior course of the main conducting bundle appear to predispose to fibrosis and the development of progressive atrioventricular dissociation even in the absence of surgical interference. Complete heart block is rare at birth, but becomes more likely with age so that presentation with intermittent complete heart block is comparatively common in the young adult. First and second degree heart block are common findings in affected children.

Wolff Parkinson White syndrome is relatively common in corrected transposition; accessory pathways have been demonstrated in both left and right atrioventricular rings, and types A and B WPW syndrome are equally common. If there is an Ebstein-type tricuspid valve, the pathway is always left sided.

Clinical presentation

While isolated congenitally corrected transposition of the aorta and pulmonary artery allows a normal circulation, 70% of affected infants present in the first year of life with significant right-to-left or left-to-right shunts, requiring surgical repair.

Presentation in adults takes the following forms:

1. Complete heart block, leading to syncope or presyncope, if intermittent, or to sudden effort intolerance if sustained. This commonly occurs around the end of the third decade, and is so characteristic that the diagnosis should be excluded in any patient of this age presenting for the first time with heart block. Insertion of a permanent pacemaker is indicated for symptomatic and prognostic reasons, atrioventricular sequential dual chamber pacing is the

mode of choice. There may be technical problems associated with finding a stable position for the ventricular lead in the smooth walled morphological left ventricle and so a screw-in lead may be preferable.

2. Left atrioventricular valve regurgitation. In the absence of major associated lesions, progressive tricuspid incompetence may result in breathlessness and fluid retention in early adult life. Since the systemic ventricle is of right ventricular morphology, it is probable that significant impairment presents at an earlier stage than a comparable lesion of the mitral valve in a normally arranged heart, and although symptomatic relief may be gained from diuretics, angiotensin converting enzyme (ACE) inhibitors, and digoxin, early surgery to repair or replace the valve is indicated.

3. Decompensation. In a patient with pulmonary stenosis and a VSD, the severity of the lesions may be balanced such that there is minor cyanosis with trivial or no left-to-right or right-to-left shunt. With age the balance may be upset in several ways:
   ○ increasing pulmonary stenosis due to degenerative change
   ○ increasing tricuspid regurgitation
   ○ systemic ventricular failure

   The timing of surgical repair in apparently balanced cases with mild cyanosis is a difficult decision, but from a retrospective review of a large series of 111 cases, Lundstrom concluded that, in contrast to those patients without significant pulmonary stenosis and VSD, cyanosed patients with atrioventricular valve incompetence could safely have surgery deferred until symptoms were severe.

4. Systemic ventricular failure. The systemic ventricle in corrected transposition is of right ventricular morphology; the impedence of the systemic circulation is much greater than the pulmonary, and the ventricle is required to perform more work than it would in the normal position. It is not clear whether ventricular failure in the absence of tricuspid regurgitation is an important clinical problem, however. There are reports of patients surviving into the sixth and seventh decades with trivial complicating lesions whose systemic ventricle obviously performs well. However there are also reports of affected patients with trivial complicating lesions, who die in early adolescence from circulatory failure, in whom systemic ventricular failure appears to be the primary cause. The more usual clinical scenario, however, is of progressive left atrioventricular valve incompetence with time, and in this situation the ventricle is clearly vulnerable, so that early surgery to prevent ventricular damage is recommended.

Diagnosis

When there is clinical suspicion of the diagnosis of corrected transposition, various investigations will confirm with increasing specificity.

Electrocardiogram

When the heart is in the normal position in the chest, the surface ECG shows left axis deviation, reversal of the usual pattern of Q waves in the precordial leads, and deep Q waves in leads 2 and AVF, because of the abnormal septal depolarization. The effects of acquired atrial dilatation, and right sided ventricular strain may appear as these secondary complications develop.

Chest X-ray

If the aorta is posterior and to the right, and there are no significant complicating lesions, the chest X-ray may be normal. However, in the usual arrangement, with the aorta anterior and to the left, the heart shadow is altered so that the left border is straight with the aortic shadow obscuring the pulmonary conus and proximal left pulmonary artery. Complicating lesions will be reflected in the X-rays; a left-to-right shunt due to a VSD causes pulmonary plethora, a right-to-left shunt due to pulmonary stenosis and a VSD causes pulmonary oligaemia, and left atrioventricular valve regurgitation causes an increase in the cardiothoracic ratio, with signs of pulmonary venous hypertension.

Echocardiogram

The diagnosis of corrected transposition is usually made echocardiographically. The diagnosis is based on demonstrating atrioventricular and ventriculoatrial discordance. If the simple rules described in Chaper 2 are followed, then the sequential diagnosis should be clear in all but the most difficult of cases.

Cardiac catheterization

With the advance of echocardiography the role of cardiac catheterization and angiography has changed. Angiographic demonstration of the intracardiac anatomy is no longer necessary, but catheterization may be required to measure the following:

○ pulmonary artery pressure and resistance in the presence of a VSD
○ ratio of pulmonary to systemic flow due to a VSD
○ pulmonary capillary wedge pressure in tricuspid regurgitation
○ gradient across the pulmonary outflow tract.

Angiography may be useful in assessing:

○ the anatomy of the VSD
○ the anatomy of the pulmonary outflow and the size of the pulmonary arteries

○ left sided ventricular function and atrioventricular valve regurgitation
○ coronary anatomy

An important practical point is that the ventricular septum is usually in the midline and so all of these features are usually best demonstrated in a straight anteroposterior ventriculogram.

Surgical management

Although there is suspicion that uncomplicated corrected transposition may have a poor prognosis, there is no place at present for prophylactic morphological repair to make the morphological left ventricle the systemic ventricle (i.e. the 'Double switch' operation). Surgical repair is reserved for the congenital and acquired complications.

The lesions commonly requiring surgery are:

○ VSD
○ pulmonary stenosis
○ tricuspid incompetence

either in isolation or together.

Summary

Corrected transposition with important associated anomalies usually presents in childhood. Uncomplicated cases may present later with heart block or left atrioventricular valve incompetence requiring conventional management. Occasionally, complicated cases present in adults with a VSD and pulmonary stenosis, in whom the lesions are haemodynamically balanced until heart block or tricuspid regurgitation supervene.

Key references

Losekoot TG, Anderson RH, Becker AE, Danielson GK, Soto B (eds) (1983) *Congenitally corrected transposition.* Churchill Livingstone, Edinburgh.

18 Coronary Artery Anomalies

In collaboration with Andrew Bishop

Introduction

Anomalies of the coronary arteries are rarely responsible for clinical syndromes in isolation. Indeed, most cases in adults will be diagnosed as an incidental finding. Isolated coronary anomalies may come to attention if they predispose to accelerated atherosclerosis, for instance, as in anomalous origin of the left coronary from the right coronary sinus, or if their location results in extrinsic compression, as when a coronary artery runs between the aorta and the pulmonary artery.

There are two important primary defects in the coronaries; when a coronary artery arises from the pulmonary artery, usually the left, there are clinical manifestations in childhood or adult life, and when the coronaries are involved in a systemic vasculitis such as Kawaski's disease or juvenile polyarteritis nodosa, clinical coronary syndromes are common.

Anomalous origin of the coronary arteries from the pulmonary artery

This was first described by Bland, White and Garland in 1933. There are under 1000 cases reported, of which the majority are the infantile type. The vessel usually arises from the left pulmonary sinus (Figure 1) although it can arise from the main and even more distally from the left pulmonary artery.

In utero the pulmonary artery blood is well oxygenated, and the pulmonary artery pressure is high, but in the infant the converse is true. The natural history is then determined by the extent of the anastomoses between the left and right coronary systems. If there are poor anastomoses the area dependent on the left coronary will become ischaemic as the pulmonary vascular resistance falls in the first few weeks of life. In this usual scenario there is angina, left ventricular failure, and ultimately, infarction. Post mortem examination in these patients

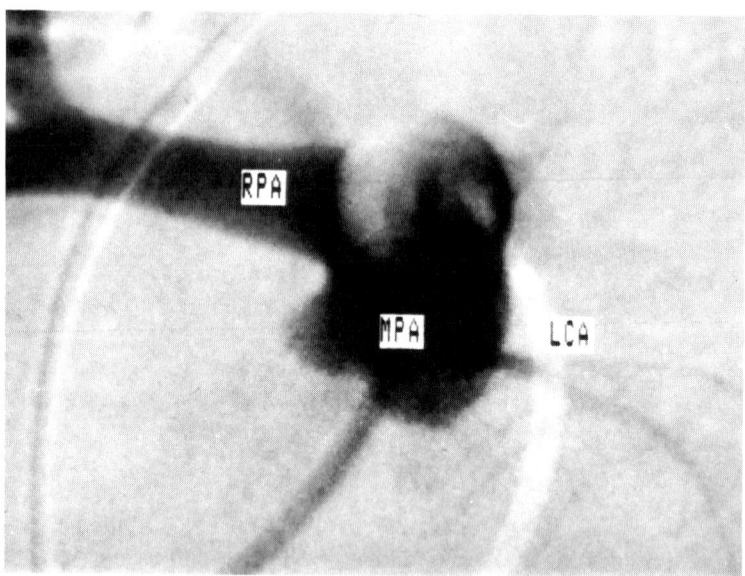

Figure 1. Subtracted balloon occlusion pulmonary arteriogram showing an anomalous left coronary artery arising from the proximal portion of the main pulmonary artery.

shows left ventricular dilatation, with thinning and fibrosis of the anterior wall and hypertrophy of the inferior wall. In some cases there are well-developed anastomoses between right and left coronaries, and blood flows through these to perfuse the left coronary territory retrogradely. Angina and left ventricular dysfunction can still develop, particularly if the flow is so large that there is steal from the capillary beds, but in a few cases virtually asymptomatic survival into adult life can occur.

Ultimately, a patient with the adult form of this condition may present with chest pain, breathlessness or arrhythmia. The diagnosis should be suspected in any patient with a continuous murmur and persistent ischaemic changes on the ECG. Thallium scanning may demonstrate regional anterior and posterior left ventricular ischaemia and echocardiography may show a dilated right coronary artery and continuous flow in the main pulmonary artery. Angiography remains the diagnostic investigation of choice, however. An injection into the aortic root will fail to demonstrate a left coronary ostium, and a right coronary injection will show a dilated vessel and may demonstrate collateral filling of the left with some late filling of the pulmonary artery. Pulmonary angiography is disappointing in showing the anomalous vessel unless the pulmonary artery is partially occluded with a balloon (Figure 1). Recently colour flow Doppler echocardiograms have been shown to be of use in distinguishing between this and other forms of dilated cardiomyopathy; retrograde flow in the left coronary, and the presence of a jet entering the pulmonary artery are diagnostic, but are best demonstrated in adults during transoesophageal echocardiography.

The treatment of this condition is surgical. Various operations are performed, but the definitive procedure, where possible, is direct reimplantation of the coronary into the aorta as first described by Neches in 1974. One occasionally encounters a patient who has undergone one of the many other procedures previously advocated in this condition:

1. Pulmonary artery banding to reduce flow from pulmonary artery to the coronary (rarely successful as pulmonary diastolic pressure remains low).
2. Aortopulmonary fistula to improve the perfusion of the left coronary with oxygenated blood (but symptons are due to low perfusion pressure, not low pO_2).
3. Ligation of the anomalous vessel to reduce both the steal and the left-to-right shunt (can be very successful).
4. Creation of a two coronary system:
    (a) anastamosis of the vessel to left subclavian or carotid;
    (b) saphenous vein graft, dacron graft, free subclavian graft;
    (c) aortopulmonary anastomosis with pericardial baffle to direct aortic blood to the left coronary.

With the exception of 1 and 2, these other approaches albeit historical, produced very good results. No matter what operation is performed the results of treatment are dependent on ventricular function, so that when there is severe left ventricular dysfunction, the prognosis for operated and unoperated patients is uniformly poor. This is contrary to the situation in young infants undergoing surgery who, despite appalling preoperative left ventricular function, have the capacity for amost complete recovery.

Coronary arteritis

In 1961 Kawasaki described the mucocutaneous lymph node syndrome in 50 Japanese children, with a peak incidence at 2 years. The disease is characterized by fever, mucocutaneous inflammation and desquamation, with conjunctivitis and arthritis. In the acute stage clinically significant carditis occurs in only 4% of patients, despite ECG abnormalities in most cases. The important lesions occur in the coronary arteries, where there is patchy inflammation of the wall leading to aneurysm formation in about one third of affected children. This can occur in epicardial and intramyocardial vessels, and favours sites of bifurcation. Interestingly, the first centimetre of each artery is often spared. In this acute phase thrombosis or rupture of an aneurysm can lead to myocardial infarction, and as in adult atherosclerotic coronary disease, left ventricular dysfunction, papillary muscle dysfunction or arrhythmia.

When the acute inflammatory phase of the disease has subsided, persistent saccular aneurysms can cause chronic angina, and are associated with left

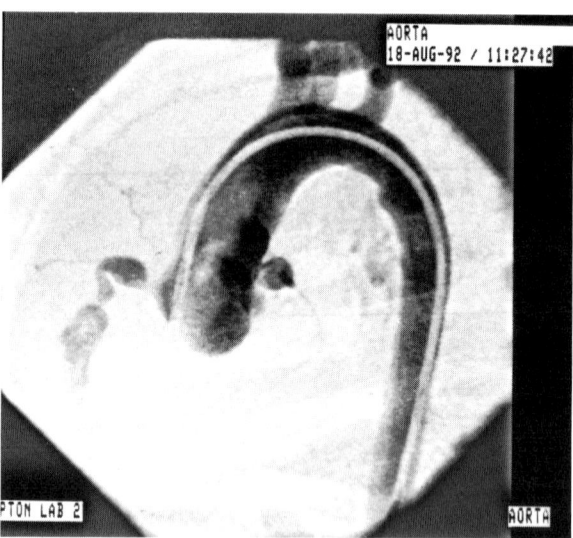

Figure 2. Subtracted aortogram from a patient 8 years after Kawasaki disease. There are saccular aneurysms of both right and left coronary arteries. The patient complained of exercise intolerance which was due to angina and left ventricular dysfunction.

ventricular disease and late sudden death, presumably as a result of ischaemia or infarction (Figure 2). Most appear to resolve spontaneously, however. Aspirin is used as an antiplatelet drug in the acute and chronic stages, and angina is managed conventionally with vasodilators and betablockers.

The prognosis for Kawasaki's disease is good with less than 3% mortality. It is unclear whether residual coronary arterial involvement is related to early atherosclerotic changes or coronary 'ectasia' seen in some young adults, but a clear-cut history of undiagnosed Kawasaki disease in childhood was given in one adult recently reported in the literature.

Congenital variations of the coronary arteries

In any sequential series of coronary arteriograms variations in the origin and course of the vessels are reported. The frequency varies with the context in which the examination is conducted, but in normal practice significant abnormalities occur in 0.1–0.5%. The anomaly may or may not have clinical consequences.

There are three sinuses in the aortic root, the right, left, and posterior sinuses, and each coronary artery has been observed arising from each sinus. In addition, the circumflex and left anterior descending arteries can arise separately, also from any sinus. More rarely the right and left coronaries arise from a common orifice (single coronary artery).

Left anterior descending artery from right sinus or right coronary artery

This pattern occurs commonly if the ventricles are inverted, and in Fallot's tetralogy (see Chapter 7); in the former the peripheral course of the vessel is mirror image. In isolation it has been associated with angina, and sudden death, and its discovery in a patient with chest pain may be an indication for bypass surgery. The more dangerous course is behind rather than in front of the pulmonary artery, since it can be compressed from behind by the aorta.

Both coronary arteries from left sinus

In this pattern, the right coronary arises anterior to the left, and runs between the great vessels. Symptoms are so rare without atheroma that it is considered to be benign.

Both coronary arteries from right sinus

This abnormality has been demonstrated at post mortem in several cases of exercise-associated sudden death. The usual course in these cases was for the left main stem to run between the aorta and pulmonary artery. The ischaemia may develop because of spasm, compression, or kinking of the vessel, or the origin of the artery may be hypoplastic or obstructed. The lesion in a young person is an indication for bypass surgery. However, when this pattern is found in adults the risk of sudden death is thought to be low, and surgery is indicated for symptoms only.

Other patterns

The circumflex artery may be absent, or arise from a separate orifice in any of the three sinuses. The right coronary may arise from the posterior sinus. The coronary ostia may lie abnormally in the sinuses, or may arise higher than the sinus. None of these patterns appear to have functional significance.

Single coronary artery

A single coronary occurs rarely in isolation, but is more common in association with some congenital cardiac lesions. In the apparently isolated cases there is an association with the presence of a bicuspid aortic valve, and the congenital lesions in which single coronary are a feature are conotruncal abnormalities, i.e. abnormalities of the ventricular outflow tracts and great vessels. These

Table 1. Classification of single coronaries (Smith, 1950)

Type 1	Single artery following the distribution of left or right coronary.
Type 2	Single artery giving proximal branches corresponding to right and left coronaries.
Type 3	Single artery with distribution different to normal left to right coronaries.

associations are a reflection of the embryological origins of the coronaries as outpouchings of the aortic root.

Single coronaries were classified by Smith in 1950 as in Table 1.

The type 3 pattern is seen very rarely except in association with other congenital cardiac anomalies. There is an increased incidence of coronary artery to ventricle or pulmonary artery fistula in all types.

Two clinical features are important. Patterns in which a major coronary trunk passes between the aorta and pulmonary artery such as origin of the left coronary from the right, are associated with sudden death, in a similar way to those with anomalous origin of the left coronary from the right aortic sinus. It is suggested that there is an increased incidence of atherosclerosis in single coronaries possibly because of increased hydrodynamic stress in long relatively unsupported vessel segments. The results of atheromatous obstruction and occlusion of a single vessel are more severe since there are no collaterals from a second system. Early surgery is therefore indicated, even in the presence of minor symptoms.

Congenital coronary artery fistula

In the embryo the developing coronary arteries are in continuity with the intramyocardial spaces that go on to form sinusoids, and persistence of these communications can lead to fistulae. The commonest sites of entry of such fistulae are the right ventricle and atrium. Less commonly there are communications with vena cavae, coronary sinus, pulmonary arteries, left ventricle, aorta or bronchial arteries. The usual form is a single fistulous tract, although multiple tracts, and plexiform connections occur. Associated dilatation and ultimately aneurysm of the feeding vessel are common.

The pathophysiological effects of the fistula depends on the its size, and the pulmonary–systemic (QP/QS) shunt that results. The mean QP/QS in a series of 74 cases reviewed by Liberthson was 1.6, and the largest reported shunt is 8.7 l/min/m^2 surface area. Accidents such as rupture or thrombosis in associated aneurysms, bacterial endarteritis, premature atherosclerosis, and direct coronary steal can lead to a spectrum of coronary syndromes from angina to infarction, left ventricular failure, and sudden death. Alternatively, the left-to-right shunt can cause fluid retention and atrial arrythmias. The diagnosis is suspected when a continuous murmur is present over the lower precordium, and angiography is the diagnostic investigation.

It is rare for the patient to remain asymptomatic in adult life, and the risk and danger of endocarditis is substantial; elective surgery or transcatheter coil embolization is therefore recommended if technically possible. Direct ligation of the tract, and repair of the associated aneurysm is the surgical procedure of choice, but complex cases may require ligation of the feeding artery and aortocoronary bypass.

Rare cases of congenital coronary artery aneurysm without associated fistula, and without a history of vasculitis have been reported, and in those cases recognized, the prognosis is poor, death occurring from rupture, thrombosis or embolism. Reparative or bypass surgery is therefore indicated.

Coronary artery patterns in congenital lesions

When there are major abnormalities of the positions and relations of the cardiac structures the course of the coronary arteries cannot be normal. The patterns of abnormality are variable even in cases with a similar underlying lesion, but two groups of conditions with similar coronary anatomy are identified.

1. Conditions where the aorta is anterior and to the right. These include transposition of the great vessels, double outlet ventricle, and rare cases of Fallot's tetralogy. In these the right aortic sinus becomes the non-coronary sinus and the posterior sinus gives rise to the right coronary. In addition the left coronary to a varying extent has common origin with the right, so that the circumflex frequently arises from the proximal right coronary, and a single coronary with branches corresponding to right and left can arise from the posterior sinus.
2. Conditions with ventricular inversion or Fallot's tetralogy. In these groups the left anterior descending artery arises from the proximal right coronary, and passes anterior to the pulmonary artery, or more rarely between the great arteries or behind the aorta. In cases of ventricular inversion, such as corrected transposition of the great arteries, the peripheral distribution of the vessels is a mirror image of the normal, so that the right coronary is conceptually a right circumflex, giving marginal branches to the anatomical left ventricle. The implication of the left anterior descending passing between the great arteries has been discussed previously.

The practical importance of understanding the arrangement of the coronary arteries in congenital heart disease is surgical. The best example of this is right ventricular outflow tract surgery in Fallot's tetralogy, where the left anterior descending artery can be damaged as it runs anterior to the pulmonary artery unless it is recognized.

Summary

Coronary artery anomalies are of minor importance in congenital heart disease, unless they result in decreased perfusion of the myocardium (e.g. anomalous origin of a coronary from the pulmonary artery), predispose to thrombosis (e.g. congenital coronary aneurysm) or premature atherosclerosis (e.g. origin of the left coronary from the right aortic sinus), or render the vessel susceptible to compression or surgical damage (e.g. the coronary patterns in Fallot's tetralogy). Surgical correction and bypass surgery are effective in the relief of angina, and in averting the risk of sudden death in those patterns with a malignant prognosis.

Section 3

Medical and Surgical Management

19 Interventional Cardiac Catheterization

In the past 10 years there has been an extraordinary expansion in the applications of various interventional techniques for the non-surgical treatment of congenital heart disease. Indeed, in some units up to 50% of catheterization procedures are therapeutic rather than diagnostic. Although specifically developed for the treatment of younger children, most of the techniques can be adapted and subsequently applied to adults with congenital heart disease. It goes without saying that these procedures should only be performed in specialized centres with appropriate facilities and expertise, but the following review will outline the indications for and some of the technical problems of these techniques in adults.

Balloon dilatation and intravascular stents

It is now possible to dilate virtually any stenosis within the cardiovascular system. The recent introduction of stent technology to improve the results of balloon dilatation of resistant stenoses has further expanded the indications for balloon dilation techniques. None the less, the primary consideration should not be whether it is technically possible to perform such techniques but whether their clinical utility, morbidity and mortality justify a non-surgical approach.

Balloon pulmonary valvuloplasty

Balloon pulmonary valvuloplasty fulfills all the criteria for a successful interventional catheterization procedure. It is cheap, safe, effective and carries extremely low mobidity and mortality. It can be performed as a day-case procedure and long-term follow up is now demonstrating that its results are comparable or superior to those obtained with surgery. There are one or two caveats, however. Failure to obtain adequate relief of purely valvular stenosis is usually due to inadequate balloon size in the adult. For a valve ring of more than 25 mm then a double balloon technique using a bilateral femoral venous approach is usually more satisfactory than a single balloon dilatation. Another possible explanation for failure is the presence of supravalve or sinutubular narrowing. This is highly resistant to balloon dilatation and although abolition of the waste during balloon dilatation can be achieved, recurrent stenosis on deflation is the norm, even when a balloon to pulmonary valve ring ratio of up to 2:1 is used. These patients will usually require surgery.

Peripheral pulmonary artery stenosis

Naturally-occurring peripheral pulmonary stenosis of the type that occurs with William syndrome, Alegial's syndrome, congenital Rubella, etc. can be very resistant to standard balloon dilatation. The same can be said of calcified circumferential anastomotic lines following surgery. None the less, this group of patients represent those with most to gain from adequate non-surgical treatment. For this reason high pressure balloons (accepting up to 15 atmospheres of pressures) and intravascular stents have been developed to overcome resistant or recurrent stenoses. Balloon-expandable and self-expanding intravascular stents have transformed the results of interventional catheterization in this group of patients (Figure 1). Satisfactory relief of peripheral pulmonary stenosis can now be achieved in up to 80% of patients, and although technically more difficult there is a low complication rate and good long-term utility. Balloon dilatation of peripheral pulmonary artery stenosis carries a significant morbidity and mortality as a result of vessel rupture. The balloon size to vessel ratio should not exceed 1:1 for the normal-sized vessel distal or proximal to the stenosis and care should be taken to avoid encroachment of the balloon into the distal pulmonary vasculature. Surgical intervention for these lesions also carries a significant risk, however, particularly in patients who have undergone multiple previous procedures, many of whom also have undergone right ventricular outflow tract or conduit surgery, and few now would recommend surgery unless an adequate balloon dilatation or stent procedure had been attempted.

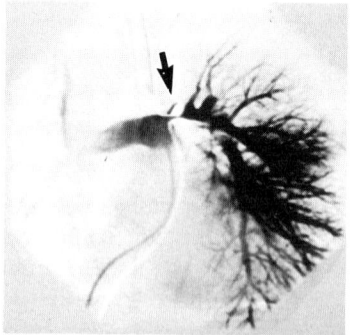 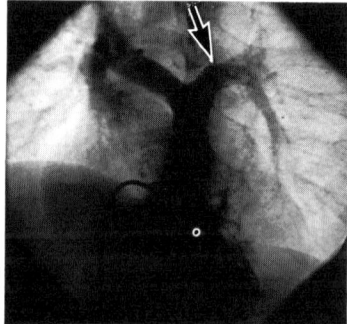

Figure 1. Severe peripheral pulmonary stenosis (arrow) after previous right ventricular outflow tract surgery (a). Balloon dilatation with placement of a balloon expandable stent (arrow) leads to complete relief (b).

Right ventricular outflow tract stenosis

Balloon dilatation of calcified conduits, xenografts or homografts is an almost futile exercise. Furthermore, dilatation of narrowed artificial conduits may lead to intimal peel and worsening haemodynamics. Occasionally, if there is discreet proximal or distal stenosis at an anastomotic line, a good result will be obtained and an individualized decision has to be made for each lesion. Intravascular stent placement across stenosed, or kinked homografts in particular, has some supporters. Relief of stenosis is at the expense of free pulmonary incompetence however, and the long-term utility of this technique remains to be seen. Unless there are pressing reasons to the contrary, we feel that homograft replacement performed by an experienced surgeon is best performed sooner rather than later.

Aortic valve stenosis

Unlike discreet subaortic stenosis, aortic valve stenosis responds well to balloon dilatation. Selection of cases is obviously important. Unicuspid or markedly disproportionate bicuspid valves can be damaged irreparably by balloon dilatation with resulting aortic regurgitation. This is less commonly a problem in adults than in neonates and infants. The ideal valve is a trileaflet non-calcified and mobile valve with normal aortic root morphology. A balloon to valve 'ring' ratio of >1:1 should never be used however. A single balloon technique is usually appropriate but the standard wire used to cross the valve should be replaced by a super stiff back-up wire to anchor the balloon across the valve during inflation, so preventing ejection of the balloon during ventricular contraction.

Adequate relief of stenosis should be achieved in the majority of suitable cases. Minor residual aortic regurgitation, or some worsening of aortic regurgitation can be expected, but rarely is it haemodynamically important. Some valves, particularly if severely fibrosed, thickened, or calcified will be resistant to balloon dilatation and will require surgery. It is not necessarily the case that a valve previously subjected to open valvotomy will not respond to balloon dilatation and dilatation of restenosis after surgery has been frequently successful in our hands.

Aortic coarctation

Coarctation of the aorta can be relieved in the majority of older children and adults by balloon dilatation. It remains an area of contention amongst interventional cardiologists however. Dilatation is achieved by dissection of the aortic wall and tears may extend through the intima and media into the adventitia of the vessel wall. As a result there is an approximate 5–10% early incidence of aortic aneurysm formation (Figure 2). Some of these will require surgical resection. The

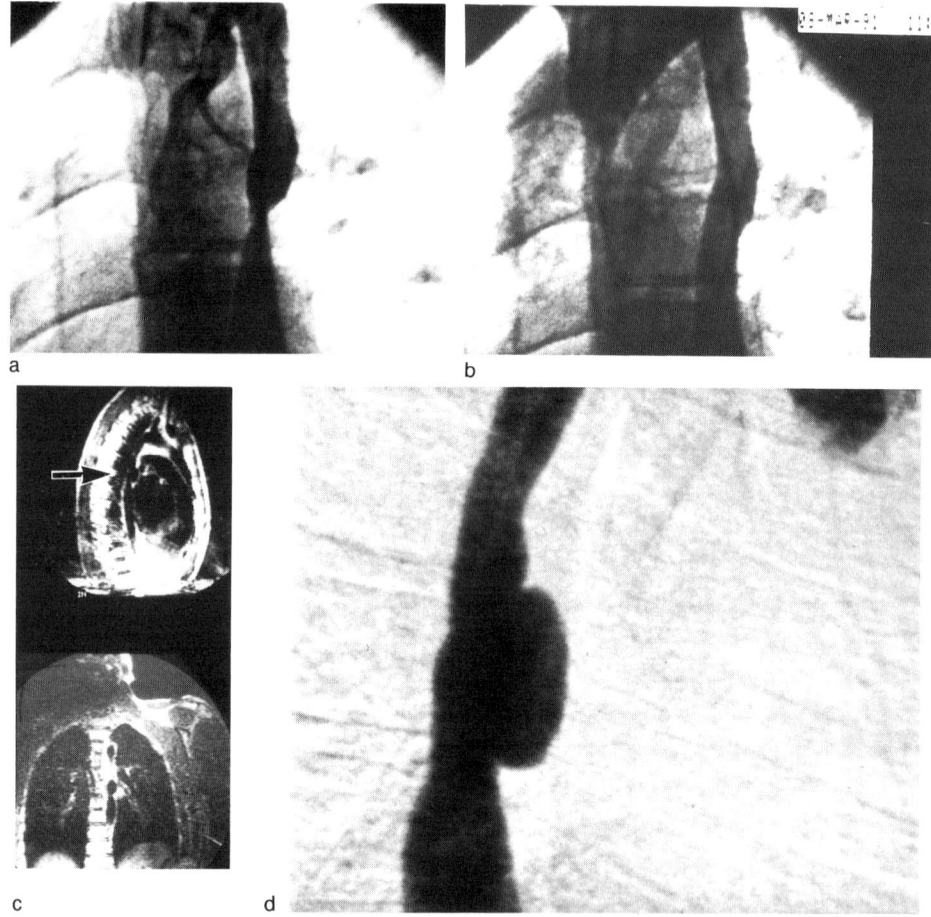

Figure 2. Angiograms showing diffuse thoracic coarctation in a patient before (a); immediately after (b); and 3 months after balloon dilation (c) shows NMR scan; (d) shows subsequent aortogram. Although complete early relief of coarctation was achieved, a saccular aneurysm developed (arrow), necessitating surgical resection.

long-term results are unknown. All patients undergoing this technique require long-term sequential reassessment, ideally with magnetic resonance imaging, although most aneurysms appear within the first year after dilatation. The antagonists to the technique further emphasize the uncertainty of the integrity of the aortic wall, particularly in women of childbearing years where hormonal changes during pregnancy may further weaken the aortic wall, and childbirth may increase the stresses on it. Its protagonists emphasize the satisfactory results obtained in the majority. For us, surgical resection with end-to-end anastomosis or subclavian flap repair is a straightforward procedure with a low morbidity and virtually zero mortality that we cannot justify the non-surgical approach. It remains popular in some units, however.

Baffle stenosis

Approximately 10–20% of patients over ten years after the Mustard operation will have significant baffle obstruction of either the superior or inferior pathways or both. Systemic venous stenosis responds well in the short-term to balloon dilatation and for many a single dilatation is all that is required. Recurrent stenosis is seen in a few, and most recently we have obtained excellent results with intravascular stent placement. Surgery is now only infrequently required. Pulmonary venous baffle obstruction is less common but more difficult to deal with. Short-term results of balloon dilatation, performed retrogradely via the aorta, right ventricle and tricuspid valve are variable but some obtain good relief. This is rarely maintained however, and most of these patients subsequently come to surgery.

The importance of post-Fontan pathway stenosis has been emphasized in Chapter 4. Where a xenograft or homograft has been placed, balloon dilatation may not be adequate for the reasons discussed above. Once again, balloon dilatation with or without stent placement has revolutionized the treatment of the majority of these patients. Reoperation carries a significant mortality (up to 40%) and it is only rarely performed. We are currently recommending that all patients receive oral anticoagulation after the Fontan procedure but this is particularly important if an intravascular stent has been placed in the pathway. Under these circumstances we vigilantly maintain an INR of between 2 and 4. This is not necessary when stents are placed in the pulmonary arteries of patients with normal right sided pressures and flow, e.g. after tetralogy of Fallot repair.

Miscellaneous

Congenital mitral and tricuspid stenosis is rarely suitable for balloon dilatation, particularly in adults. None the less, those valves fulfilling the criteria established for rheumatic mitral stenosis may sometimes be suitable for transcatheter dilatation, but this is unusual. Dilatation of shunts, e.g. classical Blalock Taussig shunt, Waterston anastomosis or aortopulmonary collaterals can sometimes be performed to good effect in those patients where improved oxygenation is required, particularly when corrective surgery is not contemplated. We have further improved the palliation of such patients by the placement of endovascular stents in for example the stenotic lower end of a classical Blalock Taussig shunt and in aortopulmonary collaterals in the setting of complex pulmonary atresia with ventricular septal defect, for example. Balloon atrial septostomy or balloon dilatation of a restrictive atrial septal defect is sometimes performed. By and large these techniques lead to partial relief rather complete relief of stenosis. If there is any doubt that residual stenosis may be haemodynamically important then surgical septectomy is usually preferable.

Vascular occlusion

Thrombogenic coils

These are used to occlude abnormal vascular structures such as aortopulmonary collateral arteries, pulmonary arteriovenous malformations, surgical shunts,

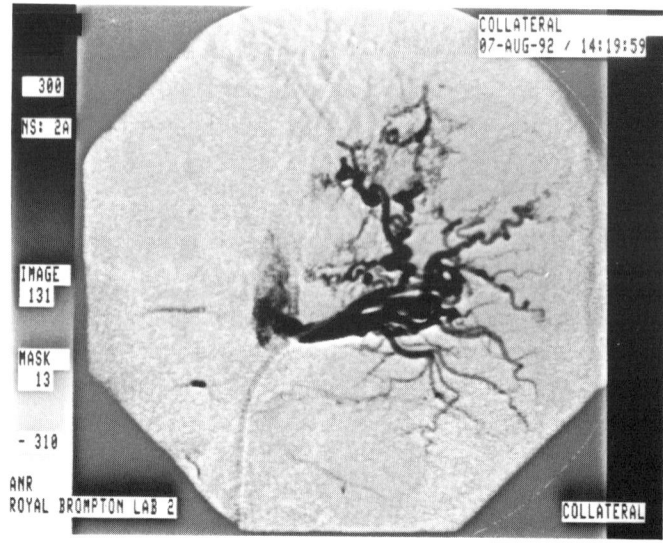

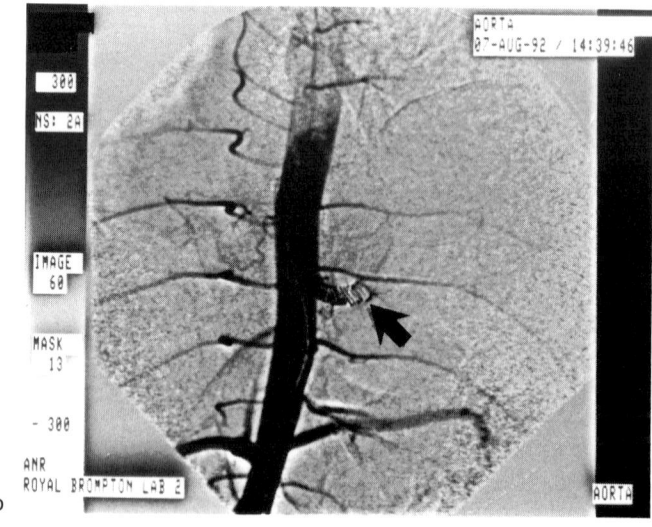

Figure 3. Coil occlusion of residual aortopulmonary collateral (a) to much of the left lung. In (b) the stump of the occluded collateral can be seen proximal to the coils (arrowed). Complete occlusion has been achieved.

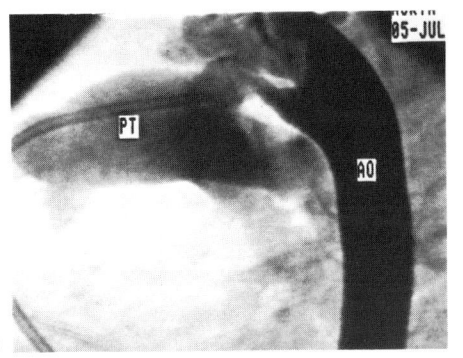
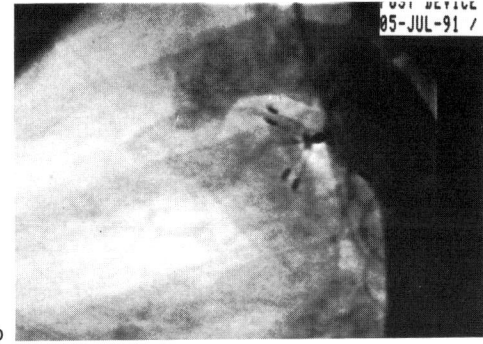

a   b

Figure 4. Umbrella closure of the adult PDA. (a) Shows the arterial duct; (b) shows the 17 mm double umbrella device across the lesion.

occasionally the arterial duct. When deployed they reform to a coiled shape but can be passed through the central lumen of a standard end-hole catheter placed in the target vessel. Their sizes vary from a few millimetres to up to 2 cm and they work by inducing intravascular thrombosis around the site of the deployed coil. They are highly effective and easy to use (Figure 3). Their complications are essentially those of distal and proximal embolization, usually as a result of poor patient selection. Distal embolization to the peripheral vascular bed may occur if too small a coil is chosen, allowing for passage through the stenosis, and proximal embolization results from attempting to place a coil in too short a proximal portion prior to a stenosis. This is a particular problem when dealing with some types of aortopulmonary collateral. Under these circumstances, an umbrella device may be more appropriate (see below).

Detachable balloons

The indications for detachable balloons and gel foam are similar to those for thrombogenic coil devices. Detachable balloons are usually filled with silicon rubber or contrast material and in the past have been somewhat unreliable because of deflation and subsequent embolization. The technology has improved in recent years however, and although rarely a technique of first choice in our catheter laboratory, detachable balloons should be available for use under specific circumstances.

Umbrella devices

The Rashkind ductal occlusion umbrella is now routinely used throughout Europe for the treatment of the arterial duct in children and has established itself as the method of first choice for the closure of the arterial duct in adult life.

Ligation of a calcified arterial duct in an older adult has a significant morbidity and mortality whereas transcatheter placement of a 17 mm umbrella device is usually straightforward and effective (Figure 4).

Although designed specifically for closure of the arterial duct, these devices have been used to occlude many intracardiac and intravascular communications. This is a specialized field and not for the faint-hearted, but we have closed naturally occurring atrial septal defects, fenestrated Fontan, ventricular septal defect, aortopulmonary collaterals, and ruptured sinus and valsalva aneurysm, in adults.

Key references

Lock JE (1991) The adult with congenital heart disease: cardiac catheterisation as a therapeutic intervention. *J Am Coll Cardiol* **18**: 330–31.

O'Laughlin MP, Perry SB, Lock JE, Mullins CE (1991) Use of endovascular stents in congenital heart disease. *Circulation* **83**: 1923–39.

20 Surgery for Congenital Defects

Introduction

Just as in children, surgery for congenital heart disease in adults may take the form of primary correction, palliative procedures in those unsuitable for primary correction, reoperation following primary correction, and occasionally transplantation.

Implicit in the title of this chapter however, is that the demands of surgery for congenital heart disease in the adult population are different from those of surgery for acquired heart disease in adults and for congenital heart disease in a younger age group.

In less developed countries primary correction of congenital heart disease in adults remains relatively commonplace. Elsewhere, with the trend towards ever earlier primary corrections, there has been a gradual reduction in the numbers undergoing primary correction in adult life. Subsequently, there has been a steady increase in the number of patients requiring reoperation following an earlier correction. In the modern era, reoperation for technical failure has fortunately become rare so that the majority are required for recurrent stenosis and regurgitation of atrioventricular or ventriculoarterial valves, prosthetic valve degeneration and conduit obstruction. They are no less challenging however. There are several important factors that significantly influence the outcome of surgery in these patients, each of which needs careful preoperative evaluation.

General considerations

Factors that predispose to an increase in mortality and morbidity after surgery for congenital heart disease in adults include:

- chronic cyanosis;
- abnormality of renal function;
- ventricular hypertrophy.

Cyanosis

Patients with chronic cyanosis bleed more than those with normal preoperative arterial saturation. This is due to two main problems; the development of profuse collateral circulation; and abnormalities of haemostasis.

Systemic to pulmonary collaterals

The presence of large aortopulmonary collaterals should always be identified by selective angiography in chronically cyanosed patients undergoing cardiopulmonary bypass. In some, they are acquired and probably derive from dilated bronchial arteries. In the majority they are integral to the underlying anomaly, e.g. complex pulmonary atresia. If the size of the central pulmonary artery and their segmental distribution is considered adequate to allow a corrective procedure, the systemic pulmonary collaterals should be embolized prior to surgery. If they are not amenable to embolization then they should be ligated before the commencement of cardiopulmonary bypass to prevent systemic arterial 'steal' and persistent 'bleedback' from the pulmonary artery. This may obscure the operative field and there is a danger of ventricular distension if the heart is inadequately vented. Indeed, hypothermia and low flow cardiopulmonary bypass may be required in some patients in order to reduce the pulmonary venous return to manageable levels.

Haemostasis

Chronic cyanosis may also lead to a derangement in haemostasis, deficiencies in platelet number and function, and abnormalities of both intrinsic and extrinsic coagulation systems with elevations of the prothrombin time and activated partial thromboplastin time have all been reported. We and others have tried preoperative phlebotomy in selected patients but the biggest impact has been made by the routine use of Aprotinin, a platelet activator, in adult cyanotic patients undergoing corrective surgery. Meticulous attention to haemostasis during sternotomy and during closure is mandatory. Fresh frozen plasma, platelets and cryoprecipitates should be immediately available and in large quantities. In our experience, the use of whole blood, platelets, fresh frozen plasma and cryoprecipitate is significantly greater in cyanotic as compared to non-cyanotic patients (Figures 1 and 2).

Renal function

Postoperative renal impairment is particularly common in this group of patients. Many have been chronically dependent on diuretics, have reduced cardiac output and may have suffered renal insults during previous surgery. The single most important factor is the presence of preoperative cyanosis however. In our

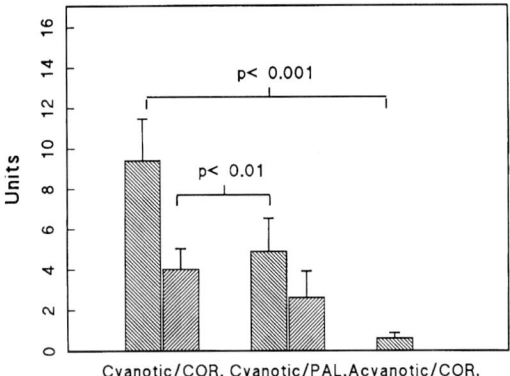

Figure 1. The average use of fresh frozen plasma (▨) and cryoprecipitate (▧) in adult patients undergoing palliative (PAL) and corrective (COR) surgery for congenital heart disease at the Royal Brompton Hospital. Significantly more is used in cyanotic patients.

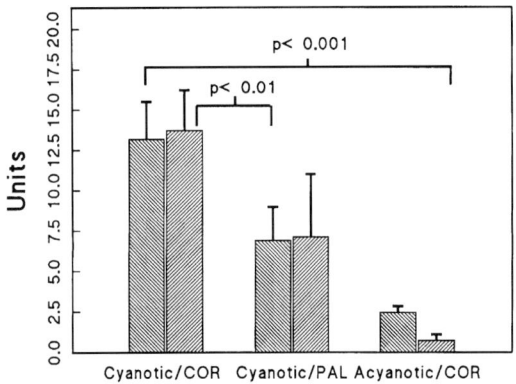

Figure 2. Blood (▨) and platelet (▧) usage is similarly higher in patients with chronic preoperative cyanosis. See Figure 1 for labels.

experience a rise in serum creatinine of 25% or more is significantly more likely in cyanosed compared to non-cyanosed patients (Figure 3). It goes without saying that meticulous attention to fluid balance and non-invasive renal support is required, but most importantly this type of surgery should only be performed when invasive renal support is readily available.

Ventricular hypertrophy and abnormalities of diastolic and systolic function

The presence of chronic pressure and volume overload lead to abnormalities of both systolic and diastolic function. The preoperative selection criteria in this regard may be quite different in adults with acquired heart disease. Right

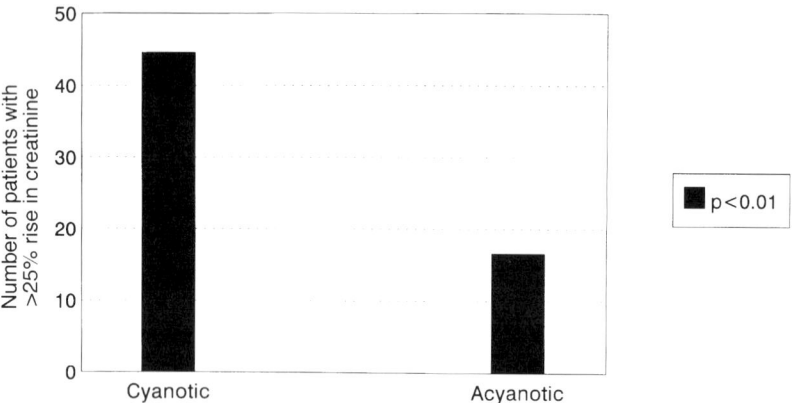

Figure 3. Significant postoperative renal impairment is more common in cyanosed patients (see text for details).

ventricular dysfunction is often the rate-limiting step in the circulation and this needs to be carefully assessed preoperatively and frequently reassessed post-operatively. The need for optimal myocardial preservation cannot be over-emphasized. We presently use blood cardioplegia usually delivered anterogradely and repeated every 25 minutes or sooner if there is a profuse collateral circulation. A left ventricular vent is inserted to avoid ventricular distension. Systemic hypothermia at 25°C is employed or at 20°C if low flow cardiopulmonary bypass is required. Residual haemodynamic defects are tolerated very poorly and careful intraoperative assessment of the repair is mandatory. Assessments include intraoperative pressure monitoring, the exclusion of residual shunting and transoesophageal echocardiography. It is worth remembering that significant shunts can occur through the large porous patches used to close VSDs in adults and we now prefer to use composite patches of pericardium and Dacron™ or a non-porous material such as Gortex™.

Reoperation

Most reoperations are performed because of degeneration of conduits and prosthetic valves or the progressive malfunction of native valves. A small number of reoperations are required for the medium or long term, and well-recognized, complications of some surgical procedures such as baffle obstruction following the Mustard procedure. Hopefully these will become less frequent as surgical techniques are improved. The timing of reoperation is one of the most difficult decisions to make in these patients but is crucial to its success as it influences not only the surgical morbidity and mortality but also the long-term result. Obstructed or regurgitant valves and conduits must be replaced before irreversible myocardial degeneration or pulmonary vascular disease occurs. It is usually unwise to wait for symptoms, particularly with right heart lesions. For example, it is now well known that the mortality for replacement of a right ventricular to pulmonary artery conduit is higher once the patient becomes symptomatic and emphasizes the need for experienced cardiological surveillance.

Preoperative evaluation: what the surgeon needs to know ——

In general, preoperative haemodynamic data is provided by cardiac catheterization or Doppler echocardiography and frequently a combination of the two. Supplementary information can be added by the use of magnetic resonance imaging. We have found this most useful in the assessment of the pulmonary trunk and pulmonary arteries to the hilar of the lungs and the assessment of the aortic arch. Indeed, with so many imaging techniques available, there can be no justification for blind or exploratory surgery. Coronary arteriography should be performed in any patient who has symptoms of, or is at risk of, ischaemic heart disease or who has poor right or left ventricular function to exclude damage to coronary arteries which may have occurred at the primary correction. In patients with tetralogy of Fallot and pulmonary atresia in particular, but any chronically cyanosed patient in general, aortography and where appropriate selection injection of aortopulmonary collaterals should be performed unless previous investigations have excluded their presence (see above).

Although we have emphasized the need for detailed morphological information, the practical importance of assessing the retrosternal space in all patients undergoing reoperation for congenital heart disease cannot be over-emphasized. Unless the position of vital structures is known, there is a real possibility of significant morbidity and mortality during opening of the sternum alone. This is best performed by magnetic resonance imaging. The position of the right atrium, right ventricle, the ascending aorta and any right ventricular pulmonary artery conduit should be carefully assessed. The close proximity of any of these structures to the inner table of the sternum, particularly in the midline, should be noted. Pressure erosion of the inner table of the sternum is a particularly ominous sign rendering resternotomy particularly hazardous. The techniques employed for reopening should take into account the risk of breaching any of these structures.

Resternotomy ——

The technique of resternotomy should be individualized. The important considerations are the assessment of the restrosternal space (see above), the presence of a ventricular septal defect, aortic regurgitation and major aortopulmonary collaterals. For example, if the right side of the heart, including a right ventricular pulmonary artery conduit is breached during resternotomy, resulting in sudden loss of blood, air may enter the heart and reach the systemic circulation through even a small ventricular septal defect. Another problem is encountered with cardiopulmonary bypass in the presence of aortic regurgitation or major aorto-pulmonary collaterals. We have already mentioned the problem of run-off reducing systemic perfusion, but if the heart fibrillates there may be severe ventricular distension and ultimately poor postoperative function. For these reasons, in all but the most straightforward reoperation, exposure of a femoral artery and vein is carried out before the sternotomy is performed. Where there is major risk of inadvertently entering the heart, femoral-to-femoral cardiopul-monary bypass with deep hypothermia to 20°C and circulatory arrest is employed prior to sternotomy. Using this technique it has proved possible to perform sternotomy and quickly dissect out the right side of the heart for bicaval cannulation using no more than 15 or 20 minutes circulatory arrest even in the presence of dense adhesions. Ventricular distension (see above) is a hazard of this technique if the heart fibrillates during cooling but this can be minimized by external cardiac massage or direct venting of the left side of the heart through the chest wall while the patient is quickly cooled to the desired temperature.

Postoperative care

The principles of postoperative care in adult patients with congenital heart disease who have undergone primary correction or reoperation are similar to those for patients with acquired heart disease, namely the maintenance of adequate cardiac output and gaseous exchange. There are specific problems encountered in this group. There were significant differences in the length of

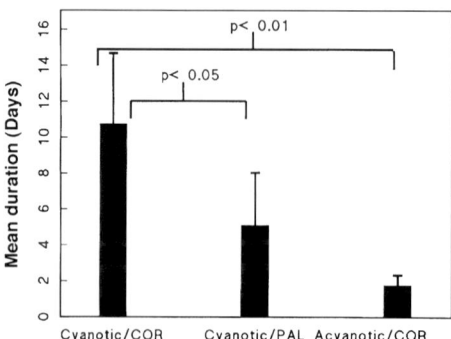

Figure 4. The increased morbidity associated with preoperative cyanosis is reflected in a significantly prolonged postoperative intensive care stay in these patients.

stay in ITU when the group with cyanosis was compared to the non-cyanotic group (Figure 4). We have already emphasized that cyanotic patients are prone to develop bleeding diatheses and abnormalities of renal function postoperatively and supportive treatment should be started sooner rather than later. Supraventricular tachycardias which may have been a cause of cardiac decompensation preoperatively may persist in the postoperative patient. These are particularly poorly tolerated in patients with ventricular hypertrophy and diastolic dysfunction and every effort should be made to restore sinus rhythm.

We consider intraoperative and postoperative transoesophageal echocardiography to be an essential part of the management of these patients. Not only does it allow rapid assessment of the surgical result, but it also identifies and follows the development of residual haemodynamic defects, systolic and diastolic dysfunction and the effects of supportive treatment with inotropes, etc.

21   Surgery

Introduction

It is estimated that in Britain (population 55 million), approximately 200 operations a year are required nationwide for treatment of congenital heart disease in the adult population. Historically the development of the cardiological and surgical management of congenital heart disease in children has been aided by the concentration of patients into the hands of a few appropriately trained and committed individuals. Worldwide the best results have been achieved where large units have developed and been appropriately staffed and funded. Because of the comparatively small numbers of adults with serious unoperated congenital heart disease and because of the exponential rise in the number of these patients requiring reoperation the arguments in favour of concentrating these patients in a small number of units is persuasive.

We have already in general terms eluded to some of the more important facets of preoperative evaluation and surgical technique. We believe that operations should be performed by personnel trained and practising in both adult and congenital heart disease and the importance of a close liaison between physicians, surgeons and interventional cardiologists cannot be over-emphasized. Balloon dilatation and stent insertion in pulmonary arteries in surgically created pathways may be either an alternative or an adjunct to reoperation. Balloon dilatation can be either a definitive treatment or part of staged management of the treatment of stenotic valves. Coil or umbrella embolization of collaterals may be either a definitive treatment for excess pulmonary blood flow or cardiac failure or a means of facilitating and reducing the risks of corrective surgery in some forms of cyanotic heart disease. The need for a close liaison between cardiologists and surgeons further strengthens the argument in favour of concentrating funds and patients.

What follows is an account of personal experience of operations performed on adults with congenital heart disease at the Royal Brompton National Heart and Lung Hospital between July 1987 and December 1993. During that period 198 patients with congenital heart disease over the age of 15 years underwent operation. Of these, 69 patients (32%) underwent surgery for a defect of the atrial septum, and 67 (50% of the remainder) were reoperations. The results, reflecting the learning curve of surgeon, cardiologist, intensivists, etc. are encouraging and perhaps not as bad as one would expect in this difficult group. Eleven patients died within 30 days of surgery producing a 30-day mortality of 5.5%. Of the 11 deaths, five patients had undergone previous corrective surgery. There is more to surgical results than 30-day mortality, however, and the individual subgroups bear closer analysis.

Atrial septal defect

The number of patients in this series undergoing a primary correction of atrial septal defect over the age of 15 years, and the type of defect is depicted in Table 1. As anticipated, by far the vast majority (56 out of 69) were of the secundum type. With contemporary clinical practice and medical screening the number of atrial septal defects requiring closure in adult life should continue to decrease. Presentation in the adult population usually occurs as the result of routine medical screening revealing the typical clinical signs or chest X-ray appearances. Alternatively patients may present for the first time when symptoms develop – usually those of shortness of breath on exertion or palpitations. In older patients the development of symptoms usually coincides with the development of an atrial arrhythmia or left or right atrioventricular valve regurgitation.

Although the clinical benefit consequent on closure of an ASD is not universally accepted, it is our experience that some patients are markedly improved both in terms of relief of symptoms and reduction in heart size. Our policy of recommending closure is supported by the low incidence of postoperative morbidity and zero mortality. In patients younger than 40 years of age and without evidence of pulmonary hypertension, the ASD can be closed without prior cardiac catheterization. In those with clinical evidence of hypertension, those over the age of 40 and those at high risk of ischaemic heart disease, cardiac catheterization should be performed to establish the pulmonary vascular resistance and to perform coronary arteriography.

As in children, ASDs can be closed by either primary suture or, if large, with a patch of autologous pericardium. If pericardium is required, the patient should

Table 1.   Operations on the atrial septum between July 1987 and December 1993

	Number of patients	Hospital deaths
Primum ASD	5	0
Secundum ASD	56	0
Sinus venosus ASD	4	0
Common atrium	1	0
Atrial septectomy	1	0
ASD & PS	2	0
Total	69	0

be anticoagulated for 3 months postoperatively as we have seen both pulmonary and systemic emboli as a result of a thrombus forming on the pericardial patch. Interestingly, these patients seem particularly prone to the development of significant pericardial effusions which can form both within days or weeks after surgery, resulting in pericardial tamponade in some cases.

Ostium primum ASD presenting for correction in adult life is usually diagnosed as a result of routine medical examination or symptoms of progressive left atrioventricular valve regurgitation. Techniques to close the ASD and correct the atrioventricular valve incompetence do not differ from those used in the children. Mitral valve replacement is rarely required for a valve which has not been previously repaired. As in all instances of atrioventricular valve repair, intraoperative transoesophageal echocardiography should be available.

Left ventricular outflow tract obstruction

Thirty-seven patients in this series underwent operations on the left ventricular outflow tract (Table 2). There were no hospital deaths.

A stenotic bicuspid aortic valve is one of the most common congenital malformations accounting for the majority of operations in this group. In patients with non-calcified valves balloon dilatation should be attempted before surgical intervention. Patients who have undergone a previous surgical valvotomy rarely have a successful outcome from a second valvotomy performed in adult life. Careful consideration should be given to the choice of prosthesis in those requiring valve replacement. The age of the patient, the likely need for reoperation, the risks of anticoagulants as well as lifestyles and the wish to bear children should all be taken into consideration. The size of the aortic root may also have an important bearing on valve selection.

In young adults (less than 35 years of age) the rapid degeneration of xenograft valves precludes their use. Mechanical valves have superior durability and the present generation of tilting disc low-profile valves have a satisfactory

Table 2. Number of operations performed for left ventricular outflow tract obstruction between July 1987 and December 1993

	Number of patients	Reoperation	Hospital deaths
Aortic valvotomy	6	1	0
AVR	14	8	0
Resection of subaortic stenosis	10	2	0
Aortic root replacement	6	1	0
Supravalvar aortic stenosis	1	0	0
Total	37	12	0
Coarctation	19	4	0

haemodynamic profile. However, even with careful control of anticoagulation, the risk of a thromboembolic event is 2–4% per patient per year to which must be added a similar risk of anticoagulant therapy.

A detailed account of the preservation of homograft valves and the effect of preservation techniques on viability and long-term function is beyond the scope of this chapter but in general terms 80–85% of patients are free from valve leaflet degeneration 10 years after valve insertion. Longer-term durability may be favourably influenced by cryopreservation and the use of 'homovital' (fresh) valves. A homograft valve in the aortic position offers the advantages of less risk of thrombocmbolism without the need for anticoagulation. They are haemo-dynamically superior to any available bioprosthesis or mechanical valve and therefore are most suitable for use in the patient with a small aortic root. Methods for insertion include subcoronary valve replacement or aortic root replacement with coronary reimplantation. Aortic root replacement may prove the most effective method of preserving the valve geometry, particularly in patients undergoing reoperation, but this is speculative.

The use of patient's own pulmonary valve as an autograft to replace the aortic valve or root, together with reconstruction of the right ventricular outflow tract by the insertion of a homograft is presently receiving widespread attention because of the almost flat survival curve for the pulmonary autograft at 20 years, demonstrated in the series implanted by Donald Ross who pioneered the technique. A register has recently been established to pool data from centres more recently adopting the use of this procedure.

Twenty-five per cent of patients in this series who had left ventricular outflow tract obstruction required relief of subaortic stenosis. The techniques employed included resection of a subaortic shelf, removal of thickened endocardium by enucleation from the left ventricular outflow tract and myectomy. For more diffuse types of subaortic stenosis, more radical procedures including aortic root replacement or patch enlargement of the ventricular septum with preservation of the aortic valve may be required.

Coarctation of the aorta

Twenty-three patients in this series underwent operation for coarctation of the aorta. Four of these patients had recoarctation. There are features of the surgery for coarctation which are of less importance in the paediatric age group but require careful management in older patients. The anatomy of the coarcted segment together with the anatomy of the aortic arch and descending aorta must be clearly defined preoperatively. In addition to angiography we have found magnetic resonance imaging often provides a clearer image of the coarctation. Because of the association of coarctation with abnormalities of the aortic and mitral valves, complete echocardiographic and Doppler assessment of intracardiac anatomy is mandatory and coronary angiography is essential in those at risk of ischaemic heart disease. Percutaneous coronary angioplasty of significant coronary lesions should be considered prior to coarctation repair.

Great care must be exercised when performing thoracotomy to avoid excessive blood loss from chest wall collaterals and large collaterals should be ligated and not diathermized. In adults great care must be taken in mobilizing the aorta below the segment of coarctation because of the presence of large, very friable collaterals. The surgical techniques currently employed for the correction of coarctation in adults include resection with end-to-end anastomosis or bypassing the narrowed segment with a tube graft between the aortic arch or left subclavian and the descending aorta. The use of patch angioplasty is avoided wherever possible because of the unacceptable risk of aneurysm formation. Use of a graft is particularly favoured for the correction of recoarctation where mobilization of the recoarcted segment may be particularly difficult.

It is important to perfuse the distal aorta in order to protect the spinal cord from ischaemic injury. This is particularly important when the distal aortic pressure falls below a mean of 50 mmHg during aortic cross clamping or when it is anticipated that the repair will require more than 30 minutes of cross clamp time. We have found heparinized shunts inadequate to reliably provide adequate perfusion pressure in the distal aorta and presently prefer to use femoral–femoral bypass. Using this protocol, only one of the 23 patients in this series developed transient minor motor weakness postoperatively which fully recovered. There were no hospital deaths.

Tetralogy of Fallot

In this series 18 patients underwent primary repair of tetralogy of Fallot and 18 patients who had undergone previous repair required reoperation (Table 3). The mean age of patients undergoing primary correction was 34 years. Patients who are well balanced because of their anatomical features or following previous palliation are recommended operation to prevent later decompensation. Other patients require operation because of progressive cyanosis, shortness of breath and decreased exercise tolerance and yet others develop cardiac failure usually coinciding with the development of supraventricular tachyarrhythmias.

Preoperative investigation and assessment of operability is dealt with in previous chapters but the size and distribution of the pulmonary arteries must be clearly defined and any distortion of the pulmonary arteries caused by a previous shunt must be evaluated. Magnetic resonance imaging as an adjunct to pulmonary angiography will aid evaluation of the pulmonary arteries. As mentioned earlier, pulmonary artery pressures must be measured when previous palliative procedures have been performed. Aortography should be performed to assess the degree of any aortic regurgitation and selective coronary angiography used to exclude the possibility of an anomalous coronary artery crossing the right

Table 3. Number of patients undergoing either primary correction or reoperation for tetralogy of Fallot between July 1987 and December 1993

	Number of patients	AGE		Hospital deaths
		Mean	Range	
Primary repair	18	36.7	14–60	1 (5.6%)
Reoperations	18	24.5	17–60	3 (16.7%)
Total	36			4 (11.1%)
		Causes of death		1. ARDS
				2. RV failure
				4. Low CO and hypoplastic LV

ventricular outflow tract and in older patients to exclude the presence of coronary artery disease.

Patients presenting for correction in adult life may have had previous palliation afforded by classical or modified Blalock Taussig, a Pott's or Waterston shunt. Any type of shunt may cause pulmonary artery distortion or narrowing requiring repair of the pulmonary artery at the time of corrective surgery. Where a classical Blalock Taussig shunt has been performed, great care must be taken in dissecting out the subclavian artery prior to bypass. The subclavian artery can be very friable and easily injured, particularly in older patients. Take-down of Pott's or Waterston shunt requires the use of cardiopulmonary bypass having established control of the pulmonary artery distal to its insertion. Profound hypothermia and low flow techniques may be required for take-down of a Pott's shunt which is most easily performed from within the left pulmonary artery.

There are a few technical points concerning intracardiac correction of tetralogy of Fallot in adults worthy of mention. The markedly hypertrophied right ventricular myocardium is difficult to retract and often hinders exposure of the ventricular septal defect. This is therefore best approached by a combined transatrial–transventricular or a transatrial–transpulmonary approach. The hyper-trophied muscle holds sutures poorly and interrupted buttress sutures should be used around the whole of the circumference of the defect. Because of the size of the VSD patch required, we prefer to use a non-porous material as significant shunting can occur through large porous patches in the immediate postoperative period. It is our experience that these hypertrophied ventricles tolerate pulmon-ary regurgitation poorly and therefore if it is necessary to perform a transannular patch to relieve right ventricular outflow tract obstruction adequately, a homo-graft valve is inserted in the pulmonary position. Residual haemodynamic defects are poorly tolerated and the repair should be evaluated by intraoperative trans-oesophageal echocardiography. Of the 18 patients in this series undergoing primary correction of tetralogy of Fallot there was one death within 30 days of surgery, attributed to hypoplasia of the left ventricle. However, the presence of preoperative cyanosis and arrhythmias, poor ventricular compliance and in some cases cardiac failure resulted in a number of postoperative complications and prolongation of ITU stay.

Reoperation following correction of tetralogy of Fallot

Eighteen patients in this series underwent reoperation following previous correction of tetralogy. The indications for reoperation included residual ventricular septal defect, right ventricular outflow tract obstruction, obstruction of a right ventricular/PA conduit and cardiac failure occurring as a result of pulmonary regurgitation.

Patients requiring reoperation for a significant ventricular septal defect in adult life after previous correction in childhood almost always have associated residual right ventricular outflow tract obstruction. Right ventricular outflow tract obstruction occurring in the absence of a ventricular septal defect and resulting in a gradient of more than 50 mm between right ventricle and pulmonary artery, require surgical relief and should be performed before right ventricular dilatation and dysfunction occur as a result.

In the long-term follow-up of patients after correction of tetralogy of Fallot, between 3–5% of patients require correction of pulmonary regurgitation. The usual indication is progressive right ventricular dilatation associated with a reduction in exercise capacity. Our policy, in these patients, is to replace the pulmonary valve with a pulmonary or aortic homograft. In a small number of patients who had previously undergone correction of tetralogy of Fallot in childhood, a right ventricular pulmonary artery conduit had been used, usually to avoid damage to an anomalous left anterior descending artery. The use of conduits in this situation has now largely been circumvented by the adoption of transatrial repair. Where conduits have been used in the past, reoperation may be required for conduit obstruction. Replacement of conduits is dealt with in the following section.

Of the 18 patients undergoing reoperation for tetralogy of Fallot there were three hospital deaths. The mortality was higher in this group than in any other diagnostic category. One patient died of adult respiratory distress syndrome and a second patient died of cerebral injury. A third patient with right ventricular outflow tract obstruction died of right ventricular failure. This patient had severe impairment of right ventricular function preoperatively, consequent on a delay in referral.

Change of conduit

The use of a conduit between the right ventricle and the pulmonary artery was first reported in 1963 by Kleiner and Zencker using a woven Teflon™ graft. A year later Kirklin reported the use of a non-valved pericardial tube, followed in 1966 by a report from Ross and Somerville on the use of the aortic homograft. The use of xenograft valves within Dacron™ tubes was first reported in 1970. The disadvantages of composite grafts formed from xenograft valves and Dacron™ conduit soon became apparent when rapid calcification of the valve was seen, particularly in younger patients. Intimal peel developed within the Dacron™ tube and both elements of degeneration conspired to produce high, early and progressive gradients. These pathological changes outweigh the advantages of these conduits over aortic or pulmonary homografts, namely availability and the fact that they are easier to remove and replace. However, there are still exponents of their use, particularly when a conduit is required in an infant when rapid growth of the patient will require their early replacement, for example in the correction of truncus arteriosus.

On the other hand the homograft has excellent long-term results; in one series of patients in which the homograft had been used as an RV/PA conduit in patients with pulmonary atresia and tetralogy of Fallot, 70% were free of reoperation for right ventricular outflow tract obstruction 20 years after insertion. The technique for their insertion is critical if such good long-term results are to be achieved. Compression behind the sternum must be avoided and the geometry of the valve must be preserved. It has also been demonstrated that the use of a Dacron™ graft to extend the length of the homograft resulted in only 52% free of obstruction 10 years after insertion.

Clearly, all patients in whom a conduit has been used between the right ventricle and the pulmonary artery need continuous cardiological surveillance. The conduit should be changed if there is a resting gradient of more than 50 mmHg between the right ventricle and the pulmonary artery. It is worthy of note that new arrhythmias are usually indicative of an adverse change in haemodynamic status although 50% of patients with severe obstruction are symptom free. Failure to deal with conduit obstruction before the onset of symptoms may prejudice both the early and late results of conduit replacement. Preoperative assessment should be made by a combination of Doppler echocardiography, angiography and magnetic resonance imaging. It is important to establish whether or not there is significant obstruction distal to the insertion of a conduit. We have already mentioned the use of magnetic resonance imaging to provide detail of the branch pulmonary arteries. Clearly any distal obstruction should be dealt with surgically at the time of conduit obstruction although the insertion of stents may be an alternative.

An important part of the preoperative evaluation includes an assessment of the retrosternal space to identify precisely the position of the conduit and its relationship to the midline and the inner table of the sternum. This is best achieved by magnetic resonance imaging. The procedure for resternotomy will depend on the perceived risk of entering the conduit and damaging the right atrium or ventricle.

We believe that exposure of the femoral artery and vein before resternotomy is mandatory. If the preoperative assessment has indicated that the conduit lies directly behind the sternum in the midline, cardiopulmonary bypass is established before sternotomy. Occasionally when there are additional haemodynamic problems, for example, ventricular septal defect or aortic regurgitation, hypothermia is established and circulatory arrest induced before resternotomy.

After resternotomy the right side of the heart and the aorta are dissected out. Both cavae are cannulated together with the aorta. The aorta is cannulated if the femoral artery has not been used. In the absence of any communication between the left and right side of the heart, the conduit can be changed without cardiac arrest. In other cases blood cardioplegia is used. A detailed account of the technique used to remove and replace conduits is beyond the scope of this chapter but it is worth emphasizing that during dissection of the conduit one must remain in the correct plane of dissection between the conduit and any overlying fibrous tissue. We have found this is facilitated by detaching the conduit proximally and dissecting it towards its distal attachment. Great care is needed, particularly when removing homografts to avoid damage to the aorta when aorta and conduit lie in close proximity. In all cases where a conduit between the right ventricle and the pulmonary artery was removed it proved possible to replace the conduit with an aortic or pulmonary homograft using a hood of pericardium to complete closure of the ventriculotomy and thereby avoiding the use of Dacron™ grafts.

Sixteen patients underwent change of conduit between the right ventricle and the pulmonary artery (Table 4). There were nine concomitant procedures including five who underwent repair of a more distal pulmonary artery stenosis. There were three hospital deaths: one patient died of adult respiratory distress syndrome; one died of right ventricular failure; one patient who underwent reoperation after a Fontan procedure for conduit obstruction died due to elevation of the pulmonary vascular resistance which occurred as a result of repeated pulmonary emboli.

Table 4. Diagnostic categories and concomitant procedures in patients undergoing change of conduit between July 1987 and December 1993

Diagnosis	Number of patients	Hospital deaths
VSD & PA	3	1 (33.3%)
Fallot's/absent PV	6	1 (16.7%)
Truncus	1	0
Fontan	3	1 (33.3%)
AVSD	1	0
Corrected TGA	1	0
Total	16	3 (18.7%)
Concomitant procedures	PA repair	5
	Correction of residual shunt	2
	AVR	1
	Enlargement of VSD	1

The Fontan procedure

The creation of an atriopulmonary connection and closure of ASD for tricuspid atresia was first described by Fontan in 1971. Since that time the Fontan procedure has been more widely applied in the surgical management of congenital heart disease to include patients with absent left connection, double inlet ventricle, hypoplasia of right or left ventricles and including those with atrial isomerism. The techniques employed for the redirection of systemic venous blood to the pulmonary arteries and the criteria considered necessary for a successful outcome have undergone continual modification. The most important considerations are the size of the pulmonary arteries, the pulmonary artery pressure and pulmonary vascular resistance and the systolic and diastolic function of the ventricles. The bidirectional Glenn and its later completion to a Fontan operation has recently been introduced as a strategy for high-risk patients, although in some centres staging of the operation is routinely used.

Although there is evidence that early mortality after the Fontan procedure is more likely in adults than in children, excellent functional results have been reported in carefully selected patients. As in other forms of uncorrected cyanotic heart disease, functional deterioration requiring surgical intervention may be required because of progressive cyanosis, shortness of breath and decreased exercise tolerance. Clinical deterioration may also occur because of progressive atrioventricular valve regurgitation, particularly in those patients with a common atrioventricular valve. Yet others will deteriorate as a result of supraventricular tachyarrhythmias which may be difficult to control medically.

The surgical technique that we currently employ for connecting the systemic venous return to the pulmonary arteries in the adult population is similar to that used in children and follows closely the technique for total pulmonary venous connection described by deLeval and others. This technique is modified to take into account anomalies of systemic venous return. In those patients with atrial isomerism, bilateral superior vena cavae and azygous continuation of the inferior vena cava, we prefer to direct hepatic venous return to the pulmonary arteries in addition to performing bilateral anastomoses between the superior vena cavae and the pulmonary arteries.

Eleven patients underwent a primary Fontan procedure, either by a direct atriopulmonary connection or by a total pulmonary venous connection. There was one death in a patient who had a borderline pulmonary vascular resistance. Only one patient underwent a bidirectional Glenn procedure as the first stage of a total pulmonary venous connection. In this patient the superior vena cava was the sole source of pulmonary blood supply, which proved inadequate: total cavopulmonary connection was successfully performed 3 weeks after the Glenn anastomosis. Because the percentage of the total systemic venous return through the superior vena cava is less in an adult than in a child we feel this may limit the use of the bidirectional Glenn as a preliminary to the Fontan operation if it is the sole source of pulmonary blood supply.

Reoperations after the Fontan procedure

Reoperation is required after the Fontan procedure almost exclusively for stenosis of the atriopulmonary connection. This is more likely to occur if a conduit is used rather than a direct atriopulmonary anastomosis. Indeed it has been demonstrated that long-term survival after the Fontan procedure is adversely affected by the use of conduits. Even a small gradient across the atriopulmonary pathway can result in a marked reduction in cardiac output and elevation in venous pressures with peripheral oedema, ascites, hepatomegaly and derangement in liver function, etc. Preoperatively these patients must be fully assessed, usually by a combination of echocardiography, cardiac catheterization and magnetic resonance imaging. It should be remembered that a measured gradient between pulmonary artery and atrium may be under-estimated in the presence of low cardiac output. Magnetic resonance imaging may detail both the site and severity of anatomical obstruction not evident on angiography. Elevation of pulmonary artery pressure may be an indication of impaired ventricular function or an elevation of pulmonary vascular resistance consequent on repeated pulmonary emboli. Systolic and diastolic function of the ventricle together with function of the atrioventricular valve should be assessed by Doppler echocardiography. It is important to remember that in the patient with a Fontan procedure and low cardiac output, more than one factor may contribute to the low output state. Revision of the atriopulmonary connection is likely to be successful if this is the only or the predominant cause. Where ventricular failure is the cause of low cardiac output, transplantation should be considered.

Deterioration after the Fontan procedure may occur late as a result of intractable supraventricular tachyarrhythmias, consequent on high right atrial pressures and right atrial distension. It is possible that such patients may benefit by conversion of the atriopulmonary connection to a total pulmonary venous connection, but this is speculative.

Four patients underwent reoperation after the Fontan procedure for change of conduit. One patient died as a result of pulmonary thromboembolic disease.

Transposition of the great arteries

Patients with transposition of the great arteries who have undergone a previous Mustard or Senning procedure may present in adult life with symptomatic deterioration. This may be caused by either stenosis of the systemic or pulmonary venous pathways or by right ventricular dysfunction. In patients with no more than moderate impairment of right ventricular function, relief of systemic or pulmonary venous obstruction can be achieved by baffle revision and/or enlargement of the pulmonary venous atrium. When severe impairment of right ventricular function is the cause of symptomatic deterioration, anatomical correction should be considered. In patients undergoing anatomical correction, preparation of the left ventricle by pulmonary artery banding is usually indicated. Alternatively these patients can be managed by transplantation, particularly if there is coexisting left ventricular dysfunction.

Five patients underwent reoperation after the Mustard procedure. Three patients had stenosis of the systemic venous pathway and two patients had stenosis of both the systemic and the pulmonary venous pathways. There were no hospital deaths.

Transplantation

Although most complex congenital heart disease can be managed by conventional surgery some patients have anatomical features precluding surgical correction. Another group of patients are those who develop myocardial dysfunction after surgical correction, e.g. after a Fontan or Mustard procedure. Patients in either group should be considered for transplantation if they remain in functional class IV in spite of optimum medical therapy and there is no other reasonable therapeutic option. Techniques of orthotopic heart transplantation have been developed to take account of cardiac position, atrial site, anomalies of systemic and pulmonary venous return and position of the great arteries.

Transplantation is possible if the pulmonary arteries are of good size and the pulmonary vascular resistance less than 6 units. Only a small series of patients undergoing transplantation for end-stage congenital heart disease in adult life have been reported, but 3-year survival as high as 80% has been achieved.

Section 4
Specific Problems

22 Pregnancy and Contraception

In collaboration with J Chambers

Introduction

The prevalence of congenital heart disease amongst women of reproductive age is increasing as improvements in paediatric cardiology prolong survival. Providing these women with sound advice about conception and contraception is essential, as both carry greater hazards than usual. Unfortunately the heterogeneity and generally small numbers of fertile women with congenital heart disease mean that little research specific to them has been performed. The family planning advice must therefore derive from this small body of data combined with a 'common sense' approach – the latter being an attempt to predict what is for the best based upon a thorough understanding of the pathophysiology of the patient, the physiology of pregnancy and the known effects of the various contraceptive measures in normal women. Armed with this information the physician can advise the woman with a cardiac anomaly what hazards pregnancy poses to her, the medical advisability of conception and the most appropriate contraceptive for her. There will, of course, be times when personal considerations outweigh such medical advice and it is worth remembering that an aspiration of medicine must be to assist these women to live as freely and fully as possible.

Pregnancy in congenital heart disease: assessing the need for contraception

For the woman with congenital heart disease pregnancy may carry significant hazard for her and/or her fetus. In these women the physician may become closely involved in the decision as to whether she should conceive, providing an assessment of the risks that pregnancy would entail and hence the advisability of contraception.

Pregnancy makes considerable demands upon the maternal cardiovascular system: understanding these can help predict and understand how a particular cardiac lesion will behave ante-, intra- and postpartum. Blood volume increases by 50% on average as a result of expansion of the red cell and plasma volumes. The latter is increased proportionately more, giving the 'physiological anaemia of pregnancy'. Cardiac output increases by about 45% during pregnancy and can increase by a similar amount again in labour. Both heart rate and stroke volume rise. Venous return also rises (except during periods of uterine caval compression), systemic and pulmonary vascular resistances fall. Left ventricular end-diastolic volume (but not pressure) increases. Atrial and ventricular ectopics become more common; sinus rhythm is otherwise well maintained. Blood pressure initially falls slightly then rises again in the last trimester. Immediately postpartum central blood volume may show marked swings – it may be increased as the contracting uterus empties of blood or decreased if there has been significant peripartum haemorrhage. Infection is a common feature of the puerperium. Pregnancy is a hypercoagulable state with venous stasis, increased clotting factors and reduced fibrinolysis.

With these normal physiological changes in mind it becomes easy to understand which cardiac lesions are likely to cause significant maternal hazard in pregnancy. Broad division into high, moderate and low risk lesions is possible.

The risk of pregnancy

High-risk lesions include pulmonary hypertension (whether primary or as part of the Eisenmenger syndrome), aortic stenosis, mitral stenosis, Marfans syndrome and any lesions giving NYHA grade IV breathlessness. The Eisenmenger syndrome is particularly dangerous, carrying a maternal mortality rate of 30–70%, mainly from either increased cyanosis or low cardiac output. The early postpartum period is a time of especial hazard (possibly in part due to sudden alterations in venous return). In congenital aortic stenosis pregnancy increases the transvalvular gradient as cardiac output rises whilst SVR falls. Similar considerations apply to mitral stenosis. For women with Marfans syndrome the dominant hazard is of course aortic dissection, made more likely both by the haemodynamic changes, but also by the hormonal effects which weaken the aortic wall.

Lesions carrying moderate risk to the mother include coarctation, cyanotic heart disease without pulmonary hypertension and prosthetic valves. Fallot's tetralogy can behave quite unpredictably with the increased venous return and systemic vasodilation causing on occasion profound hypoxia. For the mother with a prosthetic valve the dangers are of premature valve failure (biological prostheses) and thromboembolic phenomena.

Low risk lesions are fortunately the most common. Uncomplicated ASD and VSD are very well tolerated although paradoxical embolization is a potential hazard. One particular problem of the unoperated ASD and VSD occurs during labour, and delivery. Blood loss may lower right atrial pressure and lead to an increase in left-to-right shunt, 'stealing' from the systemic circulation progressively and sometimes catastrophically. Intravenous fluid replacement should be rigorously maintained in these patients. Mitral regurgitation, aortic regurgitation and pulmonary stenosis are generally well tolerated.

Fetal welfare

The above discussion relates entirely to maternal welfare, but consideration should also be given to the fetus. Particular hazards to the fetus are maternal cyanosis, maternal drug therapy, maternal requirement for cardiac operation on bypass whilst pregnant and genetic risk. Maternal cyanosis is associated with increased fetal loss, prematurity, intrauterine growth retardation and fetal cardiac and non-cardiac anomalies. The degree of risk is directly proportional to the degree of desaturation and the increase in haematocrit – fetal loss approaches 100% for the profoundly hypoxic. Maternal drugs particularly associated with fetal hazard include warfarin (fetal haemorrhage and specific embryopathy), heparin (retroplacental haemorrhage) and ACE inhibitors (neonatal renal failure, oligohydramnios, growth retardation). The antiarrhythmic drugs and diuretics seem generally safe, but experience for many is extremely limited. Bypass surgery carries a fetal loss rate of around 20%. The genetic risk to the fetus is variable; for single gene defects such as Marfans the risk of transmission is 50%, whilst for multifactorial defects such as ASD/VSD the transmission rate is 4–6% (the incidence of congenital heart disease in the general population being about 1%).

With this information, assessment of maternal and fetal hazard is possible and the woman is able to make an informed decision as to whether to opt for conception or contraception. The options for contraception are discussed below.

Contraceptive options and their suitability

In general there are five contraceptive options: sterilization, intrauterine devices, barrier, traditional and hormonal methods. Each has its own particular advantages and disadvantages which may assume especial importance when taken in the context of the woman's cardiac lesion.

Sterilization

Sterilization procedures can be applied to the woman or (less desirable) her partner and are simple, safe and extremely effective. For the woman a variety of techniques exist. They are performed under general anaesthesia and may be laparoscopic (application of a ring or clips to the mesosalpinx) or by laparotomy (most commonly Pomeroy's operation – excision of a segment of fallopian tube leaving the ends divergent). The failure rate is of the order 3–5 per 1000 cases. Male sterilization (vasectomy) is equally effective and is usually performed under local anaesthesia.

The main disadvantage of sterilization procedures is that they can rarely be successfully reversed. They are, therefore, only appropriate for the woman who has decided never to conceive. In the context of congenital heart disease this is most likely to be the woman with anomalies that carry high risk and are not amenable to surgical palliation or correction. If a future surgical procedure is envisaged then a more reversible method of contraception may be preferred. Sterilization of the male partner is an option for which similar considerations apply, but the likelihood that the man will significantly outlive the woman should be borne in mind.

Intrauterine devices

A variety of intrauterine devices (IUDs) exist – they consist of inert silastic (preformed into several different shapes) with or without 'medication' added (copper wire wrapped around the stem or impregnation with a progestogen). Their mechanism of action is somewhat uncertain but they appear to block blastocyst implantation perhaps through induction of a sterile inflammatory response, alteration of myometrial activity or endometrial biochemistry. IUDs are simple to insert (outpatients or GP surgery), simple to remove, long lasting (years) and relatively effective. The pregnancy rate is generally accepted to be 2–4 per 100 woman years.

IUDs have a number of disadvantages. Menorrhagia, intermenstrual bleeding, pain and spontaneous expulsion of the device are relatively common and will be more marked in the hypoxaemic or patient taking anticoagulants. Occasionally uterine perforation may occur. Perhaps the most serious disadvantage though, particularly in those with cardiac defects, is that IUDs predispose to pelvic infection and hence bacteraemia. Approximately 1 in 50 IUD users will develop pelvic infection (less with copper medicated IUDs) in the first year after insertion (twice the rate in non-IUD users). Endocarditis consequent upon IUD-associated pelvic infection has been reported, therefore women with congenital anomalies that carry a significant risk of endocarditis should be discouraged from IUD contraception. They are probably best avoided therefore, when there is a restrictive VSD, PDA, prosthetic valve, valved conduit or aortopulmonary shunt.

Barrier and related methods

These include the male and female condom, the diaphragm, the cervical cap and spermicidal creams. They may be used in combination.

Table 1. Failure rate of barrier contraceptives

Method	Failure rate: pregnancies per 100 woman years	
	Well motivated use	*General use*
Male condom	3	10
Diaphragm	3	18
Cervical cap	5–10	20+
Spermicide only	10	20+
Cervical sponge	No reliable information	
No contraception		80

Barrier methods all have the advantage of no adverse effects on their users and some protection from sexually transmitted disease. However they require significant patient expertise, have variable contraceptive efficacy and are not aesthetically acceptable to all. The reported failure rates are shown in Table 1.

When properly used the diaphragm and condom compare favourably with IUDs and the progesterone-only-pill in terms of contraceptive efficacy and carry less hazard. However, inexperienced or incorrect use are associated with high pregnancy rates.

Traditional methods

This term is applied to methods such as coitus interruptus and the safe period. Both have high failure rates (20–30 pregnancies per 100 woman years) and cannot be recommended as effective contraception.

Hormonal methods

Hormonal methods, in particular the oral contraceptive pill, are the most frequently used contraception in the west. There is a large literature on its efficacy and safety in this broad group but very little on the specific issue of hormonal contraception in congenital heart disease.

Hormonal methods involve the use of oestrogens (steroids that promote endometrial hyperplasia) and progestogens (promote endometrial differentiation to secretory phase). Like other steroid hormones, they both act on a wide range of tissues giving a multiplicity of effects. Both are contraceptive – oestrogens via inhibition of pituitary FSH release and progestogens via inhibition of pituitary LH release (high-dose effect) and generation of a hostile endometrium and cervical mucus (low-dose effect).

There are three major administration methods: intermittent oral oestrogen and progestogen (the combined oral contraceptive, COCP), continuous oral low dose progestogen (the progestogen only pill, POP) and administration of a depot of progestogen (intramuscular injection 3 monthly, or subdermal slow release capsules up to 5-yearly). Contraceptive efficacy is highest for the depot preparations and lowest for the POP, failure rates essentially zero and 3%, respectively. These methods are generally easy to use, although the importance of regular pill taking should be stressed, particularly for the POP whose contraceptive efficacy is seriously reduced if the day's dose is more than 3 hours late.

The range of effects of oestrogens and progestogens is large and has been well characterized. Cardiovascular effects are amongst the most important and may be particularly relevant to the woman with cardiac disease. An increased risk of venous and, to a lesser extent, arterial thromboembolism in COCP users was first detected in the 1960s and has been subsequently well validated. Deep vein thrombosis and pulmonary embolus are increased up to fourfold by COCP use. This is the result of an oestrogen-dependent increase in coagulation factors, an effect that appears to be dose-dependent and is one of the arguments for favouring low oestrogen COCPs. Arterial thromboembolism manifesting, for example, as myocardial infarction or stroke also shows an increase which is probably small, induced by both the oestrogen and the progestogen, and argues for the use of low doses of both. The mechanism of progestogenic thromboembolic disease is unclear but may be via hypertension and/or lipid changes. The newer synthetic progestogens, such as gestodene and desogestrel, may be less thrombophilic than their predecessors.

Other effects of the sex steroids include hypertension, lipid changes, a reduction in malignancy of the ovary and uterus, a reduction in benign breast disease, alteration of hepatic metabolism and menstruation. Progestogen-only therapy frequently causes marked menstrual irregularity.

In any woman who has risk factors for DVT/PE the COCP should be used cautiously. Women with congenital heart disease will fall into this category if they have any of the following: low cardiac output, raised JVP, thrombogenic surfaces, dilated cardiac chambers, reduced mobility or other cause for venous stasis. Furthermore those women for whom an embolus would cause particular trouble (notably pulmonary hypertensives and cyanotics) should avoid the COCP. If hormonal methods are to be used, then depot progestogen offers an excellent combination of safety (no oestrogen) and efficacy. The lower dose progestogen of the POP potentially has a lower arterial disease risk, but also has a much higher failure rate. If the menstrual disturbance of progestogen-only therapy is unacceptable, it may be necessary to prescribe the COCP. In this instance the lowest dosing of oestrogen and progestogen compatible with contraceptive efficacy should be used.

Many women with cardiac lesions are formally anticoagulated. It has been proposed that the COCP is safe in these women as the anticoagulation will negate the prothrombotic tendency. This has not been formally tested.

Summary

Conception and contraception frequently endanger the health of the woman with congenital heart disease. Family planning advice is therefore invaluable to her. Careful consideration of her anomalies allows assessment of the dangers of pregnancy and her requirement for contraception. There are a large number of contraceptive options each with disadvantages: sterilization is safe, effective but permanent; IUDs are contraindicated for those at risk of endocarditis; hormonal methods, particularly the COCP, should be avoided in those at risk of thrombo-embolic disease or with right-to-left shunts; coitus interruptus and related methods are extremely unreliable; barrier methods require a degree of patient expertise and commitment. The great advantage of the latter, namely the absence of systemic adverse effects, should be remembered as, with practice, they can be effective and are safe no matter what the cardiac lesion.

Key references

Braunwald E (1992) Cardiovascular diseases and pregnancy. In Braunwald E (ed). *Heart Disease: A Textbook of Cardiovascular Medicine*, 4th edn, pp. 1793–809. WB Saunders, Philadelphia.

Jesperson J, Peterson KR, Skouby SO (1990) Effects of newer oral contraceptives on the inhibition of coagulation and fibrinolysis in relation to dosage and type of steroid. *Am J Obstet Gynecol* **163**: 396–403.

Llewellyn-Jones D (ed) (1990) *Fundamentals of Obstetrics and Gynaecology*, 5th edn. Faber and Faber, London.

Lotgering FK (1992) Congenital heart disease in adolescents and adults: obstetric-gynaecologic counselling. In Hess J, Sutherland GR (eds). *Congenital Heart Disease in Adolescents and Adults*, pp. 179–86. Kluwer Academic.

Nora JJ, Nora AH (1988) Familial risk of congenital heart defect. *Am J Med Genet* **29**: 231–38.

Oakley GDG (1989) Pregnancy and heart disease. In Julian DG, Camm AJ, Fox KM, Hall RJC, Poole-Wilson PW (eds). *Diseases of the Heart*, pp. 1363–71. Baillière Tindall, London.

Pitkin RM, Perloff JK, Koos BJ, Beall MH (1990) Pregnancy and congenital heart disease. *Ann Int Med* **112**: 445–54.

Realini JP, Goldzieher JW (1985). Oral contraceptives and cardiovascular disease: a critique of the epidemiologic studies. *Am J Obstet Gynecol* **152**: 729–97.

Sbaroumi E, Oakley C (1994) Outcome of pregnancy in women with valve prostheses. *Br Heart J* **71**: 196–201.

23 Infective Endocarditis

In collaboration with Dr S Balaji

Introduction

Infective endocarditis remains an important risk factor in any person with a congenital heart defect. The possibility of endocarditis should be considered in any patient with a congenital heart disease who has an unexplained systemic illness. Antibiotic prophylaxis for procedures and high-risk situations is of great importance if the prolonged morbidity and possible mortality secondary to endocarditis is to be avoided.

Patients at risk

Table 1 lists those in whom there is no need for continuing endocarditis prophylaxis. All other patients, even those with undetected bicuspid aortic valves or mitral valve prolapse are at risk, but certain groups are particularly prone to infective endocarditis. Patients with cyanotic heart disease such as tetralogy of Fallot, with high velocity jets as from a ventricular septal defect or a regurgitant or stenotic valve, and those with artificial valves or conduits are at the highest risk.

Clinical features

It can be notoriously difficult to diagnose endocarditis in patients with congenital heart disease. This is because the symptoms and signs of infective endocarditis may be 'masked' by those of the cardiac lesion and go unnoticed until there is septicaemia, frank systemic embolization or gross immune effects of infective endocarditis. Thus, any persistent fever in a patient with congenital heart disease must arouse suspicion of infective endocarditis. Other signs may be late but

Table 1.   Patient groups in whom endocarditis prophylaxis is unnecessary

○ Post ligation or umbrella occlusion of PDA (assuming complete closure)
○ Direct closure of seccundum atrial septal defect
○ Post balloon pulmonary valvuloplasty.
○ Haemodynamically normal mitral or tricuspid valve prolapse (no murmur, no regurgitation)
○ Haemodynamically normal spontaneously closed muscular ventricular septal defect

include visceromegaly, rigors, confusion and delirium. Systemic embolization may lead to splinter haemorrhages, petechiae, stroke, haematuria (renal infarctions) and abdominal pain (splenic infarction or ischaemic gut syndrome). Pulmonary embolization may lead to pleuritic chest pain, haemoptysis and respiratory distress. These are particularly sinister features, requiring detailed investigation to exclude perivascular abscess formation. The cardiac signs may be unchanged, and cannot be relied upon. None the less, a change in character of a murmur or appearance of a new murmur may occur if there are vegetations on a valve or outflow tract.

Investigations

Detailed cross-sectional echocardiography (transthoracic echocardiography (TTE) and transoesophogeal echocardiography) should be performed by an expert. Vegetations may be found in the most unusual of places. The remainder of the work-up is no different from 'common-or-garden' SBE. The most important investigations are therefore blood cultures and a full blood count (which may show anaemia, leukocytosis or thrombocytopaenia), an erythrocyte sedimentation rate (elevated), urine microscopy (for haematuria), C-reactive protein level (elevated) and circulating immune complexes (present).

All patients with congenital heart defects and a temperature must have blood cultures performed prior to initiation of antibiotic therapy. Ideally, at least three sets of blood cultures should be taken prior to starting 'blind' therapy. As in any case of endocarditis, uncontrolled use of antibiotics may greatly confuse the issue and delay treatment with specific microbiologically targeted antibiotics with disastrous consequences.

Two-dimensional echocardiography has lead to the early identification of vegetations, abscesses and cardiac sequelae of infective endocarditis. It should be performed soon after the diagnosis is suspected and then periodically if clinical and microbiological evidence of infective endocartitis is present. If adequate images of crucial areas are not obtained by transthoracic echocardiography (for example in patients with prosthetic valves), a transoesophageal echocardiogram should be done. However, the absence of vegetations or abscesses does not rule out the diagnosis of endocarditis. Endocarditis is ultimately a microbiological and clinical diagnosis and not an echocardiographic one. Vegetations may occur on valves, on the edges of a ventricular septal defect, or on the ventricular and arterial wall at the site where the jet of a ventricular septal defect or a stenotic valve has eroded the endothelium (jet lesion). Vegetations may obstruct a valve by their location and size. Abscess formation is particularly common in these patients and probably reflects the delay in diagnosis and adequate treatment, particularly with right sided lesions. MRI and enhanced computed tomography is worthwhile in any patient that does not promptly respond to therapy. This should be specifically directed towards the demonstration of lung or splenic abscesses.

Microbiology

The commonest organisms causing infective endocarditis are streptococci and staphylococci. Blind antibiotic therapy prior to availability of blood culture results must cover these two groups of organisms adequately. However, practically any bacterium may cause infective endocarditis and an exhaustive list is beyond the scope of this chapter. Expert microbiological advice must be sought in every case. Fungi and rickettsial organisms are important causes in cyanotic and immunocompromised patients and should be kept in mind.

Therapy

Blind initial therapy should be with intravenous benzyl penicillin, flucloxacillin and gentamicin at adequate doses. Once culture and antibiotic sensitivities are known, more directed therapy is started. Single drug therapy is generally not used on the basis that the organism may develop resistance. While in practice combining a bacteristatic drug may impede the activity of a bactericidal drug, this is rarely a clinical problem. Minimum inhibitory concentration (MIC) and minimum bactericidal concentration (MBC) are estimated by culturing the organism in the presence of the patients' serum. A serum level at least five times the MIC is maintained if possible. Intravenous therapy should be continued for at least 4–6 weeks, longer if artificial material (patches/conduits) is actively involved by the infection.

Role of surgery

Surgery is relatively contraindicated during the acute phase of infective endo-carditis. However, in the following situations it becomes unavoidable:

1. Severe haemodynamic compromise. Acute erosion of a valve may lead to severe regurgitation and consequent haemodynamic compromise. This is particularly true if the aortic or mitral valves are involved. A vegetation that obstructs a valve orifice or outflow tract with consequent deterioration of cardiac output may need to be removed.
2. A pedenculated vegetation of the left side which has a high risk of systemic embolization may need removal.
3. Drainage/removal of abscesses, particularly within the lung or adjacent to pulmonary arteries.
4. Unremitting infection of artificial valves, conduits and patches. Such foreign objects may need to be removed and replaced before adequate control of the infection can be achieved.

In general, at least 48 hours of adequate antibiotic therapy should be given prior to elective surgical intervention. However, the risks and benefits have to be weighed carefully in each individual case.

Prevention

A clear cause of bacteraemia prior to infective endocarditis is recognized in about two-thirds of the cases. Apart from intravenous drug users, the mouth, particularly during dental procedures, remains the main portal of entry of the organism. Good care of teeth and gums and regular visits to the dentist are the best way to prevent infective endocarditis. Antiobiotic prophylaxis is indicated for all dental procedures where the blood–mucosa barrier is breached and for all operative procedures. Early antibiotic therapy of superficial wound infections is also recommended. The need for prophylaxis for transoesophageal echocardiographic examinations is discussed in chapter 3.

Specific recommendations

For all dental procedures not performed under general anaesthesia, amoxycillin 3 g orally one hour prior to the procedure is given. Patients allergic to penicillin should receive clindamycin 600 mg orally one hour prior to procedure.

In patients having general anaesthesia 1 g intravenously is given at the time of induction of anaesthesia. In those allergic to penicillin, teicoplanin 400 mg intravenously is given at induction.

For high risk patients, i.e. those with artificial valves or conduits, ampicillin 1 g intravenously and gentamicin 120 mg (or 2 mg/kg) are given intravenously at induction followed by ampicillin 400 mg 6 hours later. If a high-risk patient is allergic to penicillin teicoplanin 400 mg (or 6 mg/kg) intravenously and gentamicin 120 mg (or 2 mg/kg) is given at the time of induction.

Conclusions

Infective endocarditis is a preventable and treatable cause of morbidity and mortality in grown-up patients with congenital heart disease. Proper dental hygiene, prophylactic use of antibiotics, and early recognition with appropriate treatment of infective endocarditis can significantly improve the prognosis in these patients.

Key references

Endocarditis Working Party of the British Society for Antimicrobial chemotherapy (1990) Antibiotic prophylaxis of infective endocarditis. *Lancet* **1**: 88–89.

Report of a Working Party of the British Society for Antimicrobial Chemotherapy (1985) Antibiotic treatment of streptococcal and staphylococcal endocarditis. *Lancet* **2**: 815–17.

Shulman ST, Amren DP, Bisno AL et al (1984) Prevention of bacterial endocarditis. A statement for health professionals by the committee on Rheumatic fever and infective endocarditis of the Council on cardiovascular disease in the young. *Circulation* **7**: 1123A–27A.

24 Exercise and Training

In collaboration with Dr S Cullen

Introduction

Although exercise is of benefit to most adolescents and young adults with congenital heart disease, some guidelines are necessary as to the sensible level of exercise that should be undertaken (Tables 1 and 2). One cannot be too dogmatic, however. There are clearly grey areas where several factors influence the level of participation in exercise, and the generally small risk has to be weighed against the desires of the patient.

Exercise capacity may be diminished in many adolescents and young adults with congenital heart disease even after surgical intervention. There are many possible reasons for this. They include: (i) inability to increase heart rate appropriately, e.g. after atrial surgery or due to medication such as beta-blockers; (ii) inability to increase myocardial contractility appropriately; (iii) inability to maintain cardiac filling pressure, e.g. after the Fontan procedure; (iv) psychological factors and habitual lack of exercise. In addition, medications may affect any recommendations concerning exercise. Those taking anticoagulants should avoid sports involving bodily contact. Patients on beta-blockers may have limited exercise capacity. In addition impaired vital capacity and respiratory function may be secondary to thoracotomy for surgical correction of heart defects.

General recommendations are given in the tables, but some specific disorders warrant some discussion.

Non-cyanotic congenital heart disease

Left-to-right shunt

In general, cardiac lesions associated with mild current ventricular (ASD, VSD, duct) volume overload are usually associated with good exercise tolerance and no risk. Similarly, individuals who have undergone corrective surgery for intracardiac

Table 1. Safe Conditions: No limitations needed

○ Left-to-right shunts, normal ventricular function
○ Mild semilunar valve stenosis
○ Mild atrioventricular valve stenosis (regurgitation)
○ Postoperative patients with normal haemodynamics

Table 2. Conditions where moderate or strenuous exercise should be avoided

○ Moderate to severe pulmonary vascular disease
○ Hypertrophic cardiomyopathy
○ Severe semilunar valve stenosis
○ Severe atrioventricular valve regurgitation
○ Exercise-induced ventricular arrhythmia
○ Postoperative patients with residual haemodynamics mimicking conditions above

left-to-right shunts, usually have normal or near normal exercise tolerance. Furthermore, the risk of exercise-induced postoperative arrhythmia is low. Occasionally patients are encountered with evidence of significant ventricular dysfunction in whom exercise capacity may be diminished and over-exertion best avoided. In general, however, all forms of exercise may be undertaken without restriction in patients who have undergone corrective surgery.

Valve stenosis

Severe or critical aortic or pulmonary valve stenosis may be associated with sudden death on exercise, and firm advice regarding activities is needed prior to relief. The need for restriction in exercise for patients with less severe aortic valve stenosis is much debated. In most cases with mild to moderate aortic stenosis, left ventricular ejection fraction is normal. Ventricular hypertrophy is not usually a contraindication to non-competitive exercise but some have suggested that regular exercise may accelerate its development. There are few data to support this, however. It seems sensible to avoid extremes of exercise in those patients with more than moderate aortic valve stenosis, particularly to curtail strenuous isometric exercise such as weight-lifting. Patients with mild or moderate pulmonary valve stenosis tolerate their lesion well and rarely have any impairment of exercise capacity. No restrictions are necessary.

Coarctation of the aorta

In some patients with coarctation of the aorta resting hypertension may persist after surgical repair or exercise testing may reveal a very abnormal response in terms of blood pressure. Aggressive treatment of resting and exercise-induced hypertension is needed before participation in sports can be recommended.

Others

Several other conditions are recognized as causes of sudden death on exercise in young adults. Hypertrophic cardiomyopathy is one of these. The risk of exercise in these patients has not been stratified either by Holter monitoring or exercise testing, and the cause of sudden death is unknown. Arrhythmia secondary to exercise-induced subendocardial ischaemia or abnormal sympathetic nervous response to exercise have been postulated, but neither has a specific reliable treatment. Abstention from competitive or strenous sports is recommended for most patients with hypertrophic cardiomyopathy. Exercise-induced ventricular tachycardia is the cause of death in some adults with prolonged QT syndrome. Again, abstinence from moderate or strenous exercise is recommended.

Patients with Marfan syndrome, with normal dimensions of the aortic root for age and size, usually have good exercise capacity with a little additional cardio-vascular risk. Competitive sports should be avoided if significant aortic enlarge-ment is present. However, regular social exercise may be undertaken with little risk.

Cyanotic congenital heart disease

Patients with uncorrected cyanotic heart disease usually have a limited exercise capacity. Cyanosis usually increases on exercise, and the secondary polycythaemia and associated hyperviscosity further impairs oxygen delivery to the exercising muscles. Although their exercise intolerance may be marked, there is little risk associated with it, and most patients can be allowed to exercise within their own limitations.

Following repair of tetralogy of Fallot, exercise tolerance is usually well preserved. Surgical residuae such as ventricular septal defect or significant pulmonary regurgitation may impair exercise capacity. Indeed, it is becoming increasingly clear that important pulmonary regurgitation and its consequent right ventricular dilatation and dysfunction can impair exercise capacity. Ventri-cular arrhythmias are particularly common following repair of tetralogy of Fallot but sudden death is rare even in long-term follow-up series. There is no evidence to suggest a link between exercise and sudden death in these patients. Unless ventricular tachycardia is consistently induced by exercise, no restrictions should be enforced.

In patients surviving into adulthood who have undergone inter-atrial repair in early childhood for complete transposition of the great arteries, exercise capacity is frequently reduced, especially at maximum levels. This may be due to inability to increase stroke volume and/or heart rate appropriately. Late impairment of right ventricular function will also play a part. Tachycardia is not well tolerated in these patients particularly if there are disturbances of atrial rhythm. Most patients can participate readily in regular social exercise. A reduction in exercise capacity necessitates a complete haemodynamic re-evaluation to assess ventricular function and to exclude venous pathway obstruction. No long-term follow-up data are available yet in patients undergoing arterial switch operation. Excluding major postoperative morbidity, e.g. myocardial ischaemia, it is hoped these patients should have a normal exercise capacity and no restrictions placed on participation and sports.

Patients who have undergone some form of Fontan operation, usually in the setting of a functionally single ventricle consistently have diminished exercise capacity. This may be a consequence of inability to increase their stroke volume and heart rate appropriately. In other patients systemic ventricular failure occurs with time and this, of course, affects exercise tolerance. Atrial arrhythmias are poorly tolerated by the Fontan circulation and strenous effort should be made to preserve normal sinus rhythm in all these patients. In general, patients following a Fontan operation should be encouraged to participate in regular social exercise but strenous sporting activities should probably be avoided. As with all other congenital heart lesions, patients tend to find their own appropriate level of exercise which they can tolerate.

In established pulmonary vascular disease exercise capacity is limited. An acute reduction in pulmonary blood flow may occur secondary to right-to-left shunting during exercise and is associated with risk of sudden death. All but modest forms of active exercise should be discouraged.

Training and cardiac rehabilitation

The cause of reduced exercise tolerance in patients with congenital heart disease may be both physical and psychological. Abnormal cardiopulmonary responses to exercise and inefficient peripheral musculature may contribute. Lack of habitual exercise and training may account for the greater reduction in exercise tolerance than one might expect for the given lesion. There is now increasing interest in cardiac rehabilitation in patients who have undergone surgery for congenital heart lesions and attention has been paid to training programmes in adults with coronary arterial disease which have led to improved exercise tolerance. The aim of cardiac rehabilitation is to improve aerobic fitness and to assess the appropriate level at which particular patient can participate in exercise. Aerobic exercises lead to an improved uptake of oxygen, whilst combinations of isometric and isotonic exercise may improve the ability of skeletal muscles to perform physical work. Perhaps more importantly, improved psychological adjustment may result from the support and encouragement provided by such training programmes. Several studies have documented significant improvement in oxygen consumption, cardiac output and duration of exercise time in children who have undergone congenital heart surgery for tetralogy of Fallot, transposition of the great arteries and other cardiac lesions.

Summary

A knowledge of the patient's clinical condition and underlying cardiac lesion is a prerequisite to offering recommendations on the safe level of participation in exercise and sports. It is difficult to make dogmatic recommendations about exercise in those who suffer from congenital heart disease. The majority of adolescents and young adults with congenital heart disease know when they need to stop during exercise and sports. There is only a minority of patients in whom abstinence from exercise should be advocated whilst the majority should be actively encouraged to take part in regular exercise.

Key references

Bradley LM, Galioto FM, Vaccaro P, Hansen DA, Vaccaro J (1985) Effect of intensive aerobic training on exercise performance after surgical repair of tetralogy of Fallot or complete transposition of the great arteries. *Am J Cardiol* **58**: 816–18.

Cullen S, Celermajer D, Deanfield J (1991) Exercise in Congenital Heart Disease. *Cardiol Young*, **1:** 129–35.

James FW, Kaplan S (1982) Ad Hoc Committee on Exercise testing, American Heart Association Council on cardiovascular disease of the Young: Standards for exercise testing in the paediatric age group. *Circulation* **66**: 1377A–97A.

25 Pulmonary Vascular Disease

In collaboration with Dr S Kaddoura

Introduction

Pulmonary vascular disease (PVD) remains as a serious complication in adults with a wide range of congenital heart defects, and leads to significant morbidity and mortality. The presence and severity of PVD has important implications for the surgical and medical management of these individuals.

This chapter deals with the clinical features, pathophysiology and management of PVD and of its consequences, including the treatment of polycythaemia, the role of oxygen, anticoagulants and other drugs, and the indications and contra-indications for transplantation. Special emphasis will be paid to the patient with severe PVD and the 'Eisenmenger reaction'. This term describes the situation where a large defect exists at the level of the ventricular septum (VSD), aorta (patent ductus arteriosus, PDA) or atrial septum (ASD), allowing free communication between the systemic and pulmonary circulations, with a balanced bidirectional or a predominant right-to-left shunt. Right-to-left shunting occurs as a consequence of a greatly elevated pulmonary vascular resistance (PVR), reaching the level of the systemic vascular resistance (SVR) or higher, and is itself a result of long-term transmission of systemic arterial pressure and increased flow to the pulmonary circulation.

Historical background

The case of a 32-year-old man with a large VSD, cyanosis, clubbing and breathlessness since childhood was described by the German physician Victor Eisenmenger in 1897. The patient had remained active until the age of 29 when he developed right heart failure and died three years later following a large haemoptysis. Post mortem examination revealed a large (2.5 cm) VSD, equally thick-walled right and left ventricles, and thick-walled atheromatous pulmonary arteries with multiple thromboses leading to pulmonary infarctions.

Table 1. Congenital cardiac lesions associated with pulmonary vascular disease and leading to the Eisenmenger reaction

---

Shunts at ventricular level
  any condition with a non-limiting VSD
Shunts at aortic level
  Large patent ductus arteriosus (PDA)
  Aortopulmonary window
  Truncus arteriosus
  Complex pulmonary atresia with large systemic collaterals (patchy)
  Postsurgical (secondary to overlarge shunt)
    Potts (descending aorta to left pulmonary artery)
    Waterston (ascending aorta to right pulmonary artery)
    Blalock Taussig (subclavian artery to pulmonary artery)
Shunts at atrial level
  Atrial septal defect (ASD) – primum, secundum, sinus venosus
  Total or partial anomalous pulmonary venous drainage
  TGA with ASD (may be early; aetiology uncertain).

The classic work of Paul Wood published in 1958 followed an 11-year study of 127 patients at the Brompton Hospital and helped to elucidate the pathophysiology and natural history of pulmonary vascular disease in adults with congenital heart disease. Wood first suggested that the Eisenmenger reaction can occur with defects at other than ventricular level. Table 1 shows the range of congenital cardiac defects which may be associated with PVD.

Pathophysiology

There are four main mechanisms leading to PVD and pulmonary arterial hypertension in adults with congenital cardiac lesions:

1. Increased pulmonary blood flow with transmission of systemic pressures to the pulmonary circulation.
2. Pulmonary vascular obstruction associated with *in situ* thrombosis and/or thromboembolism.
3. Hypoxic vasoconstriction.
4. Increased pulmonary venous pressure, for example due to associated mitral stenosis, cor triatriatum, etc.

The first of these factors is probably the most important but they often coexist in an individual, and all result in an elevation in pulmonary vascular resistance. The chronic transmission of systemic arterial pressures to the pulmonary circulation causes progressive histological changes in the pulmonary vasculature which ultimately become irreversible. This pulmonary vascular obstructive disease raises the pulmonary vascular resistance to systemic levels or higher, and makes the subsequent surgical closure of the defect hazardous and undesirable. The small muscular pulmonary arteries show the most striking anatomical changes, the severity of which has been graded as:

1. Muscular hypertrophy of the media and the development of longitudinal muscle fibres.
2. Intimal cellular proliferation.
3. Intimal fibrosis with narrowing of the vessel lumen.
4. Dilatation with thinning of the vessel wall.
5. Plexiform vascular lesions form, possibly as a result of recurrent thrombosis and recanalization and formation of new anastamotic vessels.
6. Fibrinoid necrosis of the intima and media.

Grades 1–3 are considered reversible features, while 4–6 are irreversible.

Clinical relevance and calculation of pulmonary vascular resistance

The concept of alterations in pulmonary vascular resistance (PVR) is essential and of particular interest in adults with congenital heart disease. In many such patients, when one is weighing up the pros and cons for surgery, the height of the PVR is often a critical factor. The presence of significant PVD is a contra-indication to surgical closure of a defect such as a VSD, ASD or PDA. Closure may result in death from right heart failure if the right ventricle is unable to cope with the high pulmonary vascular resistance. Careful measurement of the PVR is even more critical when assessing a potential Fontan circulation (see Chapter 10) Measurements of pressure and flow derived by cardiac catheterization (see below) are combined to calculate the PVR (mean pressure drop across the pulmonary vascular bed divided by blood flow). In health, the PVR is so easily varied that the vessels can allow the passage of 5–30 l/min without significant change in the pressure gradient across them. In the normal subject, the pulmonary artery mean pressure is approximately 15 mmHg, the atrial mean is 5 mmHg, and so the pressure difference across the lungs is 10 mmHg. If the normal flow is 5 l/min, then the resistance will be $10/5 = 2$ units of resistance. In an adult with an Eisenmenger VSD, the mean pulmonary artery pressure may be as high as 100 mmHg, the mean left atrial pressure 5 mmHg, and the pulmonary blood flow reduced to 3 l/min. This will give a resistance of approximately 32 units.

It is important that there is a normal PCO_2, plasma hydrogen ion concentration, and plasma viscosity as any elevation may significantly raise the PVR. It is also important to assess potential reversibility of pulmonary hypertension. The most commonly used agent is oxygen. In any patient with a high PVR the effect of inhalation of 100% oxygen should be measured before concluding that the resistance is fixed. Indeed, inhalation of 100% oxygen may produce such a significant fall in PVR to influence the decision on corrective surgery in the occasional patient.

Clinical features of the Eisenmenger reaction

The clinical features are similar irrespective of the site of the shunt, although PVD usually develops later in patients with atrial septal defects (ASD) than with the defects at other sites. The clinical features are to a large part the consequence of polycythaemia and hypoxaemia.

Pulmonary vascular disease is progressive and usually starts in early childhood. Some factors predispose to the early development of PVD and include Down's syndrome, associated left heart lesions such as mitral stenosis and regurgitation, coarctation of the aorta, recurrent chest infections, perinatal asphyxia and birth at high altitude.

Exertional dyspnoea is related to the degree of hypoxaemia and is more severe and occurs earlier in Eisenmenger VSD than in Eisenmenger PDA, suggesting that the symptom is related to cerebral oxygen delivery. Haemoptysis is a worrying symptom and may be small and recurrent, due to pulmonary thrombosis, thromboembolism with infarction or to haemorrhage from small plexiform vascular lesions, or it may be massive and fatal due to pulmonary arterial rupture. Haemoptysis is rare before the age of 20 and increases with age; in Wood's series, it affected 33% of all patients studied and affected all the patients who reached the age of 40. Remediable causes such as left atrial obstruction or pulmonary infection, especially endocarditis and mycetomas should always be excluded.

Exertional angina, which is probably related to an imbalance in right ventricular oxygen supply and demand, affects 15–20% of patients with Eisenmenger's reaction but is rare before the age of 20, as is exertional syncope. Sinus tachycardia on exertion occurs at all ages but supraventricular tachycardias occur with increasing frequency over the age of 30. Arrhythmias are commonest in association with atrial shunts. The onset of atrial fibrillation leads to a rapid deterioration and can be very difficult to manage. Right heart failure is a late complication affecting particularly patients in their 40s or older and is often secondary to an atrial arrhythmia or tricuspid regurgitation, which itself is rarely severe before the late 20s or early 30s. The management of these symptoms and the specific features of polycythaemia are discussed in detail below.

Clinical examination

Central cyanosis occurs and is more marked on exertion. It can be 'differential' in Eisenmenger PDA, where only the lower limbs may be cyanosed. Clubbing of the fingers and toes is a feature, but again, with Eisenmenger PDA, it may be 'differential' and affect the toes only. There may be a large 'a' wave in the jugular venous pressure due to forceful atrial contraction in the face of right ventricular hypertrophy. Clinical signs of pulmonary hypertension include a right ventricular heave, a loud and often palpable pulmonary sound (P$_2$) and a pulmonary systolic click. There may not be a murmur. The murmur of a VSD will disappear as the right and left ventricular pressures equalize. Similarly, the classical PDA murmur tends to shorten to a soft systolic murmur, and then disappear as the pressures in the pulmonary artery and aorta equalize. However, in older patients there may be murmurs of acquired tricuspid regurgitation and pulmonary regurgitation.

Chest radiograph

The main and proximal branch pulmonary arteries will be large and there may be 'peripheral pruning'. In older patients, usually past the third decade, there may be vascular calcification of a duct, a postsurgical shunt, or in thrombus or atheroma. Cardiomegaly can occur but is not invariable.

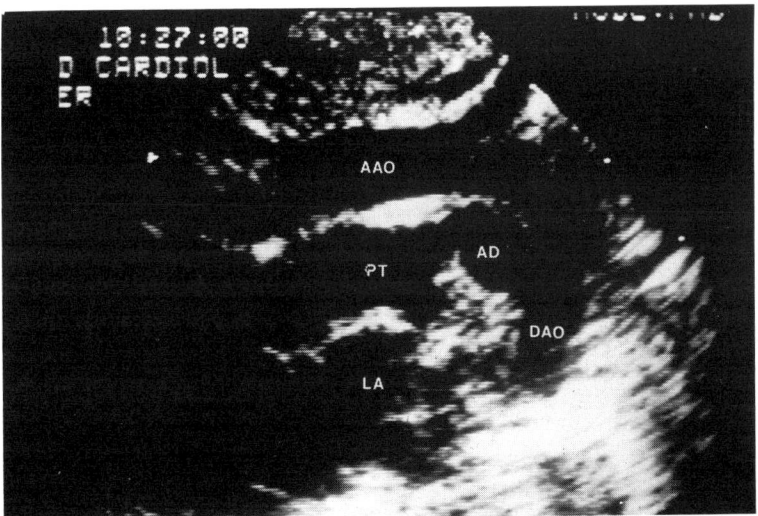

Figure 1. Cross-sectional echocardiogram in high parasternal position from a patient with differential cyanosis (pink hands, blue feet). There is a massive arterial duct (AD) with resulting pulmonary vascular disease. Consequently there is a right to left shunt from the pulmonary artery to the descending aorta (DAO). PT, pulmonary trunk; AAO, ascending aorta; LA, left atrium.

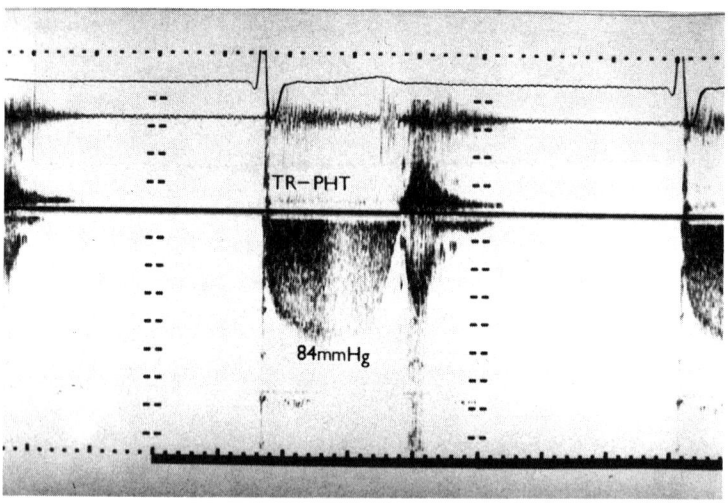

Figure 2. Doppler-detectable tricuspid incompetence from a patient with pulmonary vascular disease. The gradient between right ventricle and right atrium in systole is 84 mmHg suggesting a pulmonary artery pressure in excess of 90 mmHg.

Electrocardiogram

Right ventricular hypertrophy, right atrial enlargement and right axis deviation are typical and become more prominent with age.

Cross-sectional echo Doppler

Important anatomical and functional information can be obtained non-invasively by cross-sectional echocardiography (Figure 1) and Doppler techniques (see Chapter 2). This includes the site and size of a defect, associated anatomical abnormalities, and an indication of ventricular function. Associated tricuspid regurgitation and/or pulmonary regurgitation can be detected, enabling respectively an estimate of pulmonary artery systolic pressure and diastolic pressure to be made (Figures 2 and 3).

Cardiac catheterization

This is more hazardous in the context of PVD, particularly when relatively large volumes of contrast are used. This is because contrast agents can result in pulmonary vasoconstriction, systemic hypotension and arrhythmia. Contrast

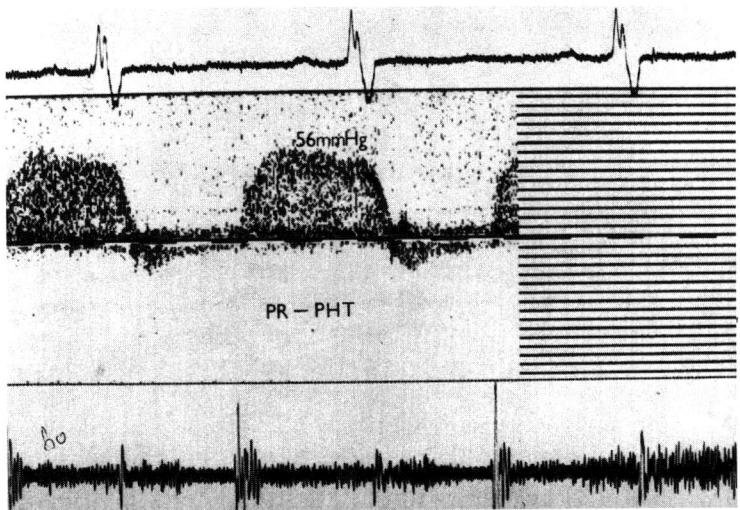

Figure 3. Pulmonary regurgitation signal from a patient with an Eisenmenger VSD. The diastolic gradient between the pulmonary artery and right ventricle is almost 60 mmHg, reflecting a very high pulmonary vascular resistance.

injection directly into the hypertensive pulmonary artery is particularly hazardous, and is rarely justifiable. Despite its risks, cardiac catheterization is required if: (i) the diagnosis is uncertain; (ii) a potentially correctable lesion such as mitral stenosis, cor triatriatum or pulmonary vein thrombosis which may increase resistance to pulmonary flow and increase right-to-left shunting cannot be ruled out using less invasive techniques, or (iii) careful, direct calculation of the pulmonary vascular resistance and its reversibility with oxygen is important when surgical options are being contemplated. Pressure measurements should be made in the main and branch pulmonary arteries, aorta and ventricles as well as directly in the left atrium whenever possible. If the left atrium cannot be entered a simultaneous measurement of pulmonary artery wedge pressure and left ventricular end-diastolic pressure should be taken to rule out left ventricular inflow obstruction. If the calculated PVR is borderline, then it is important to assess the effect of breathing 100% oxygen (see above). It is important to remember to include the effects of dissolved oxygen when calculating the PVR under these circumstances.

Natural history

Most patients with pulmonary vascular disease do well into their 20s, but often become increasingly symptomatic in their 30s. In Wood's series, the average life expectancy was 33 years for patients with either Eisenmenger VSD or Eisenmenger PDA, and 36 years for those with Eisenmenger ASD. The maximum age reached was 55 years in patients with a duct and 65 years in individuals with either an underlying VSD or ASD but this must to some extent relate to the size of the lesion and the shunt. It remains to be seen whether heart–lung transplantation will significantly affect the outcome of this group of patients, but is increasingly being performed.

The main causes of death in the Eisenmenger reaction are as follows:

1. Right heart failure.
2. Sudden, probably related to arrhythmia.
3. Haemorrhage and thrombosis: Massive haemoptysis or bleeding at other sites (related to polycythaemia and anticoagulants).
4. Infective: cerebral abscess and very rarely infective endocarditis.
5. After cardiac and non-cardiac surgery, including induction of general anaesthesia, and related to invasive cardiac investigations.
6. Pregnancy.

Specific management points and advice to patients

Since pulmonary vascular disease probably dates to early childhood, the ideal aim is to prevent its development by the early treatment of the underlying conditions listed in Table 1. By the time patients reach adulthood, pulmonary vascular disease is usually irreversible and medical treatment is mainly symptomatic.

Polycythaemia

This is secondary to a compensatory increase in circulating erythropoietin as a response to chronic hypoxaemia. The clinical features result from hyperviscosity, hypervolaemia and hypermetabolism, and are as follows:

1. Headaches and dyspnoea, both worse with exertion. Blurred vision, 'muzziness', pruritis and night sweats also occur.
2. Plethoric appearance – 'ruddy' cyanosis, conjunctival suffusion and retinal venous engorgement.
3. Haemorrhage (e.g. cerebral, gastrointestinal, uterine) and thrombosis, both venous (e.g. deep/superficial leg veins, portal, hepatic) and less often arterial (e.g. cerebral, cardiac, peripheral).
4. Gout.
5. Peptic ulceration (in 5–10%).

Venesection

The severity of the problems listed above related to the degree of polycythaemia, i.e. to the haemoglobin (Hb) concentration or to the haematocrit or packed cell volume (PCV). Venesection aims at both symptomatic relief and at reduction in morbidity and mortality; but in itself may be hazardous. It is very easy to kill a patient by badly managed or over-enthusiastic venesection. Little and often with repeated venesection of 500–1000 ml at intervals of several weeks or months, depending upon the individual patient, is the mainstay of successful treatment. The patient often knows symptomatically when it is time for a further venesection. When polycythaemia is severe (PCV>65%) a 10% reduction in haemotocrit results in up to a 38% increase in systemic blood flow, 23% decrease in systemic vascular resistance and 20% increase in systemic oxygen transport. The ideal Hb concentration to aim for is 17–18 g/dl (equivalent to a PCV of 51–54%, the conversion factor being approx $\times$ 3), although this can be hard to achieve. In patients with Hb concentrations above 23 g/dl, it is dangerous to reduce acutely the Hb to less than 20 g/dl, and no more than a 10% reduction in PCV should be attempted at any one time.

The main indications for venesection are listed below:

1. For the rapid relief of symptoms of polycythaemia. This lasts for weeks or months. There is often an increased sense of well-being, appetite and exercise capacity and a reduction in headaches and dyspnoea.
2. If the PCV exceeds 65–70% (Hb>23 g/dl).
3. To correct coagulation abnormalities (e.g. vascular thrombosis).
4. Before surgical/invasive procedures to reduce the risk of thrombosis after the procedure.

Method of venesection

The patient should be well rested for a few hours. Peripheral venous access should be obtained with a careful sterile technique to avoid subsequent sepsis. *It is vital that venesection of whole blood is accompanied by the simultaneous replacement of an equal volume of colloid,* either as fresh frozen plasma or as 5% albumin. This cannot be over-emphasized as loss of circulating volume can lead to catastrophic haemodynamic collapse.

The whole blood volume to be removed (vol) is calculated as:

$$\text{Vol (litres)} = \text{Body mass (kg)} \times 0.11 \times \frac{\text{initial PCV} - \text{final PCV}}{\text{initial PCV}}$$

where 0.11 is the estimated blood volume as a proportion of body volume. Initial PCV − final PCV should not exceed 10%.

Thus, for a 60-kg patient with an initial PCV of 80% and aiming for a 10% reduction, 0.825 litre (825 ml) should be removed over a period of at least 1 hour with continuous and contemporaneous intravenous fluid replacement, while monitoring pulse and blood pressure.

Haemoptysis

There is no effective medical treatment, other than supportive measures such as cough suppressants and antibiotic treatment of chest infection. If there is definite evidence of peripheral venous thrombosis then treatment aimed at this is indicated. Some advocate therapeutic embolization of bleeding points related to systemic–pulmonary collaterals when these can be demonstrated. Recurrent large haemoptysis is an indication for considering heart–lung transplantation.

Anaemia

Paradoxically, patients with PVD can become *relatively* anaemic despite a tendency to polycythaemia. The diagnosis is easily missed, as an Hb of 15 g/dl, for example, may be too low for adequate tissue oxygen delivery in a hypoxic individual, and can result in fatigue, anorexia, dizziness or heart failure. It can be difficult to balance the adverse effects of significant anaemia with the benefits of a lower haematocrit. The anaemia is often due to iron deficiency related to repeated venesection, but other causes of iron, folate and B12 deficiency such as menorrhagia, poor diet or pernicious anaemia should always be remembered. All patients should have a yearly blood film, looking for microcytosis or macrocytosis, serum iron, iron-binding capacity, ferritin and B12, red cell folate and a reticulocyte count. Treatment is aimed at the underlying cause, and in patients with a poor dietary intake, multivitamin supplements and a combined iron and folate preparation, should be given.

Bleeding disorders and hypovolaemia

Bleeding abnormalities are common and relate in large part to the abnormal platelet function and clotting factor deficiencies associated with polycythaemia and hypoxaemia. Correction of these abnormalities may require fresh frozen plasma, whole blood or platelet transfusions. These should always be available in any perioperative period (see Chapter 20).

Hypovolaemia due to bleeding (including inadequate fluid replacement during venesection), severe diarrhoea or vomiting can be fatal and should be managed in hospital.

Gout

This is reported in 5% of patients, as compared with 0.3% in the general population. It is related to increased red blood cell turnover in polycythaemia. The main treatment is to control polycythaemia. Colchicine is useful during acute attacks (non-steroidals should be avoided because of the risk of bleeding) and prophylactic allopurinol should be given to those with recurrent attacks. Drugs such as thiazide diuretics which increase the serum urate level should be avoided (amiloride and spironolactone are useful alternatives).

Angina and myocardial infarction

Angina is frequently improved by venesection. Vasodilators such as nitrates and calcium channel blockers should be avoided (see below). Myocardial infarction has been reported in young patients, related to hyperviscocity and thrombosis.

Heart failure

Right heart failure is a common cause of death and is often precipitated by atrial fibrillation, supraventricular tachycardia or tricuspid regurgitation. Restoration of sinus rhythm, oxygen, diuretics and inotropes are important factors in management. Severe heart failure which is resistant to conventional therapy may be an indication for heart–lung transplantation.

Syncope and sudden death

Patients should be advised to avoid strenous exercise. Exertional syncope can be related to a fall in SVR, causing increased right-to-left shunting and cerebral hypoxia, or to an arrhythmia. The latter possibility should prompt ambulatory electrocardiographic monitoring in an effort to detect a treatable arrhythmia. Sudden death, probably due to an arrhythmia, is the leading mode of death in Eisenmenger's reaction and is reported at frequencies of 14–47% in a number of series.

Cerebrovascular accident

This can occur as either a thrombotic or haemorrhagic complication or may be related to a paradoxical venous embolism due to right-to-left shunting. Management is along conventional supportive lines and with active physiotherapy and rehabilitation when appropriate. The diagnosis of cerebral abscess should always be borne in mind, and a contrast-enhanced CT brain scan is rarely contra-indicated (see below).

Cerebral abscess

This diagnosis can be missed with fatal consequences. It is probably due to 'paradoxical embolism' of bacteria due to right-to-left shunting and should be suspected in any cyanosed patient who develops any symptoms or signs that suggest meningism or raised intracranial pressure, such as headache, vomiting, fever, neck stiffness, photophobia, altered personality, decreased level of consciousness, numbness or weakness.

A contrast-enhanced CT brain scan is the investigation of choice, and treatment is by surgical drainage and appropriate intravenous antibiotics.

Skin sepsis

Acne is a common problem and is often widespread and pustular. It is related to arterial hypoxaemia. Septic foci should be treated with antibiotics, particularly prior to any planned surgery, to reduce the risk of systemic sepsis. Long-term tetracycline therapy may be used for severe cases.

Dental sepsis

Gum disease is associated with polycythaemia and central cyanosis and results in tooth loss and infection. This necessitates careful attention to dental hygiene.

Infective endocarditis (see Chapter 23)

Although the risk is low, antibiotic prophylaxis should be given for all procedures likely to be associated with bacteraemia, such as dental surgery, endotracheal intubation or genitourinary surgery.

Oxygen therapy

This is vital during the recovery from any surgery, for in-hospital treatment of severe heart failure, at high altitudes or in unpressurized aircraft (see below) and during a pregnancy proceeding to term.

The role of chronic domiciliary oxygen therapy is less clear-cut. Some patients find symptomatic relief of dyspnoea and feel more energetic with domiciliary oxygen used intermittently or for up to 15 or 18 hours daily, although there is rarely any objective evidence of improved exercise capacity. The situation has to be judged on its individual merits, following careful assessment in hospital, and oxygen should ideally be prescribed on an objective basis and not for a placebo effect.

Anticoagulant therapy

There is no firm evidence that long-term oral anticoagulation with warfarin is beneficial. The same is true of aspirin and dipyridamole. While seeking a reduction in the thrombotic complications of polycythaemia, such as cerebro-vascular thrombosis, the increased risk from haemorrhagic complications such as haemoptysis, to which these patients are also prone, probably outweighs the benefits.

Low-dose intravenous heparin may be used with careful monitoring in hospital for the acute management of thrombotic or embolic complications, but this is also not without risk. Subcutaneous and intramuscular routes of administration should be avoided as they may result in large haematomas which are uncomfortable and can become infected.

Inotropes and Vasodilators

While inotropes are invaluable in the treatment of severe heart failure in hospital, usually in patients awaiting heart–lung transplantation, there is currently no useful oral inotrope available. The indiscriminate use of vasodilators such as calcium channel blockers should be avoided. They all lower the systemic as well as the pulmonary vascular resistance and this can have disastrous consequences resulting from worsening of the right-to-left shunt. Some patients are symptomatically improved however, and if considered, treatment should be started in hospital.

Pregnancy and contraception (see Chapter 22).

Pregnancy is contraindicated and is associated with a high incidence of early spontaneous abortion and very rarely results in the birth of a healthy child. Maternal mortality in late pregnancy and the postpartum period is high, 30% in some series and as high as 60% in patients with an Eisenmenger VSD. Pregnancy is ideally prevented but termination at an early stage is probably safer for the mother despite a quoted mortality of 7% for this procedure alone.

If pregnancy proceeds to term, a vaginal delivery should be planned, with high-dose oxygen therapy, avoidance of dehydration and systemic hypotension and careful management of arrhythmias. Epidural anaesthesia is safer than a general anaesthetic for complicated deliveries.

Neither oestrogen nor progesterone oral contraceptives should be used because of the risk of thrombosis. Intrauterine devices should be avoided because of the risk of bleeding and endocarditis. Sterilization by tubal ligation is considered by most as the safest method.

High altitudes and air travel

The partial pressure of inhaled oxygen decreases with altitude, and patients with the Eisenmenger reaction should avoid altitudes in excess of 1000 m (approx 3200 feet) without inhaled oxygen therapy.

Flights in unpressurized light aircraft should also be avoided unless supplementary oxygen is available. Most commercial airliners are maintained at a cabin pressure equivalent to sea level when flying up to 6700 m (22,000 feet). When flying at higher altitudes, for example 10,000 m (approx 33,000 feet), the pressure is maintained at 2300–3000 m (7500–10,000 feet). Patients on these long, higher altitude flights (such as transatlantic crossings) should have oxygen therapy during the flight. Details of the flight should be checked in advance with the airline. Arrangements can be made in advance with many commercial carriers for oxygen to be provided.

Extra time should be allowed for travel, particularly to reduce the stress and fatigue experienced in most airports!

Exercise and sexual activity (see Chapter 24)

Patients should be encouraged to lead active lives, including engaging in sexual activity if so desired. Specific advice is difficult, but most patients are able to regulate their level of activity to a level below that which causes symptoms.

Surgical options

In patients with the Eisenmenger reaction, neither surgical closure of the shunt nor orthotopic cardiac transplantation are possible for the reasons already discussed. While in a small proportion of patients with pulmonary vascular disease, pulmonary thromboembolectomy is an option, heart–lung transplantation now offers the best hope for a cure in carefully selected patients, and this will be considered briefly.

Table 2. Contraindications to heart–lung transplantation

Malignancy
Active infection (esp. pulmonary Aspergillosis)
Hepatic or renal dysfunction (clearance <50 ml/min)
Severe chest deformity
Previous pleurectomy or major lung resection
HIV/Hep B or Hep C positive serology
High-dose steroid therapy
Uncontrolled multisystem disease, e.g. diabetes mellitus
Active peptic ulceration
Substance abuse
Uncontrolled psychiatric disease
Moribund state
Peripheral vascular disease
Age >50

* These are relative and each patient should be carefully assessed on an individual basis.

Heart–lung transplantation

Since the first successful human heart–lung transplant was carried out at Stanford University in 1981, an increasing number of patients with Eisenmenger's reaction have undergone this procedure. The results are still far less encouraging than for heart transplantation, particularly in those who have undergone previous surgery. The 4th International Registry in 1987 reported a 55% 1-year survival and a 52% 2-year postoperative survival in patients undergoing heart–lung transplantation for all conditions but is lower in those with congenital heart disease. Unfortunately, resources are limited, primarily by the lack of suitable donors, and so there are strict selection criteria which are regularly reviewed and vary from centre to centre. Table 2 shows some important contraindications to heart–lung transplantation. Some are more important than others, but they are relative and each patient should be assessed on an individual basis.

When should an individual patient be referred for heart–lung transplantation? The main indications for transplantation are on symptomatic grounds and aim to improve quality of life and prognosis in those with significant disability resistant to conventional therapy and who have an estimated life expectancy of under 18 months.

That having been said, one should not wait until the patient's clinical condition has severely deteriorated before making a referral for transplant assessment. It is often preferable to refer a patient for earlier rather than later assessment as they may have to join a sizeable transplant waiting list. The indications for transplantation are shown in Table 3.

Assessment for transplantation is a multidisciplinary process, involving not only physicians and surgeons but also nurses, dentists, physiotherapists and clinical psychologists. The rigours of the procedure itself, rehabilitation,

Table 3.   Indications for transplantation in pulmonary vascular disease

○   End-stage pulmonary vascular disease (symptoms)*
○   Frequent haemoptysis
○   Syncope at rest
○   Severe hypoxaemic angina
○   Intractable arrhythmias
○   Severe right heart failure resistant to conventional therapy

* The rate of symptomatic deterioration is important, as for example, in a patient who deteriorates from an active lifestyle to being housebound due to worsening symptoms in a period of a few months.

immunosuppression and its monitoring as well as a frank discussion of early surgical risk, have to be explained to the patient and their families.

Summary

Most individuals with pulmonary vascular disease remain active into their 20s and 30s but then become progressively more symptomatically limited. The key to maintaining a good quality of life is usually careful attention to polycythaemia and hypoxaemia. Heart–lung transplantation may offer some hope in some cases.

Key references

Gallucci V (ed) (1991) *Lung and Heart–Lung Transplantation.* Piccin, Padua.
Graham TP Jr (1987) The Eisenmenger syndrome. In Roberts WC (ed). *Adult Congenital Heart Disease.* FA Davis, Philadelphia.
Kirk AJB, Richens D, Dark JH (1993) *A Manual of Cardiopulmonary Transplantation.* Edward Arnold, London.
Miller GAH, Anderson RH, Rigby ML (1985) *The Diagnosis of Congenital Heart Disease.* Castle House Publications.
Rosenthal A, Nathan DG, Marty AT *et al* (1970) Acute haemodynamic effects of red cell volume reduction in polycythaemia of cyanotic congenital heart disease. *Circulation* **42**: 297–307.
Somerville J (1987) Congenital heart disease in adults. In Weatherall DJ, Ledingham JGG, Warrell DA (eds). *Oxford Textbook of Medicine, 2nd edn* (1987). Oxford University Press.
Wallwork J (ed) (1989) *Heart and Heart–Lung Transplantation.* WB Saunders, Philadelphia.
Wood P (1958) The Eisenmenger syndrome. *Br Med J* **2**: 701–09; 755–62.

26 Postoperative Arrhythmias

In collaboration with Dr S Cullen

Introduction

Advances in medical and surgical treatment of congenital heart disease have led to the survival of an increasing number of adolescents and young adults with simple and complex cardiovascular abnormalities. Consequently, late cardiac arrhythmias are an increasing clinical challenge to physicians who look after these patients. As a general rule, the more complex the congenital heart defect and the required surgical intervention, the greater the likelihood of important late cardiac arrhythmias and the greater the potential impact of those arrhythmias on the patient's health. Thus whereas atrial arrhythmias may be well tolerated following surgical closure of an atrial septal defect, the effect on the Fontan circulation may be devastating. The finding of a new arrhythmia in a post-surgical patient warrants a complete clinical and haemodynamic assessment.

Atrial arrhythmias

Simply stated, the more extensive and complex the surgical manipulation of the atria the greater is the tendency to develop late atrial arrhythmias. For instance, symptomatic atrial arrhythmias are unusual after repair of atrial septal defect and are usually well tolerated whereas they are a major cause of late morbidity and mortality following interatrial repair for transposition of the great arteries, e.g. Mustards/Sennings, and even more so in the various modifications of the Fontan circulation, e.g. atriopulmonary and total cavopulmonary anastomoses.

Atrial septal defect (see Chapter 11)

In the majority of cases, atrial septal defects detected in early life are electively closed before the age of 5–6 years. Early mortality is very low and long-term survival has proved to be normal. Several studies using ambulatory electrocardiographic monitoring have shown that a high percentage of post-operative patients have asymptomatic supraventricular arrhythmias, up to 80% in some reports. However, results from studies of normal populations frequently reveal the presence of similar arrhythmias whose clinical significance is unknown. Symptomatic supraventricular arrhythymia is an important although infrequent late complication after surgical closure of an atrial septal defect, occurring in less than 10%. Residual right atrial distention and right ventricular dilatation have been implicated in the causation of atrial arrhythmias.

Transposition of the great arteries

Two surgical options are available for the treatment of neonates with complete transposition of the great arteries. The current fashion is to perform the arterial switch operation wherever possible. The alternative is the well-established intra-atrial repair by Mustard/Senning procedures. Whereas detailed long-term follow-up is awaited for survivors of the arterial switch operation, late arrhythmia and sudden death are widely recognized after intra-atrial repair. Late arrhythmias include loss of sinus rhythm and the development of supraventricular tachy-cardias, especially atrial flutter (Figure 1). The extensive intra-atrial surgery involved provides the electrophysiological substrate for later development of arrhythmias which tend to be progressive. The cause–effect relationship between later arrhythmia and sudden death has been examined recently. In one long-itudinal study, 250 consecutive patients undergoing Mustard procedure for simple transposition of the great arteries were followed for up to 24 years. The risk of loss of predominant sinus rhythm (nodal rhythm) remained constant throughout the period (2.4% per year). Atrial flutter occurred in 36 of 249 patients. Furthermore, the risk of developing subsequent atrial flutter was doubled ($P<0.05$) in those with nodal rhythm, and the instantaneous risk for late death increased by a factor of almost 5 after an episode of atrial flutter (see Figure 1). The occurrence of nodal rhythm alone and importantly, functional status had no significant predictive value. Atrial flutter is an important marker of poor outcome in these patients and when diagnosed warrants a complete haemodynamic and electrophysiological investigation particularly to detect venous pathway obstruction and/or right ventricular dysfunction.

Fontan circulation

Normal sinus rhythm is essential for maintenance of adequate cardiac output in most patients following the Fontan operation or its modifications.

A

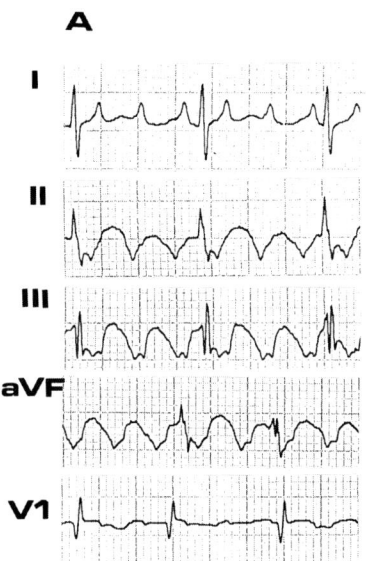

B

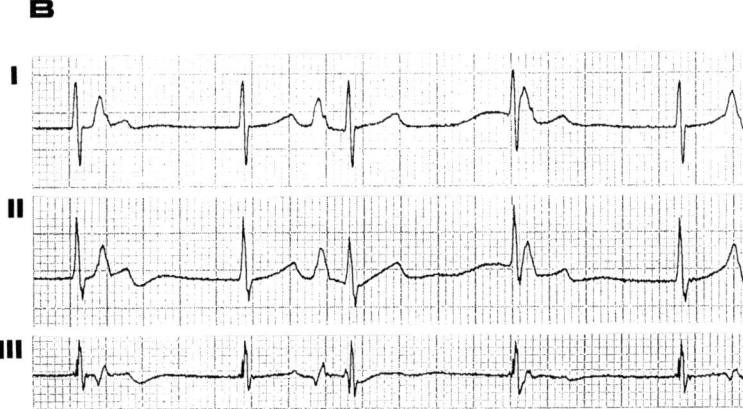

Figure 1. Sinoatrial disease after the Mustard procedure. (A) Shows atrial flutter in the same patient, a poor prognostic feature requiring careful haemodynamic and electrophysiological reassessment. (B) Shows sinus node dysfunction with escape-capture atrial bigeminy.

Atriopulmonary or total cavopulmonary connections are the most frequently employed techniques. Extensive atrial surgery is a feature of both and there is an inevitable increase in central filling pressures and both predispose to supraventricular arrhythmias. Detailed late follow-up studies are not yet available, but the preliminary data suggest that the total cavopulmonary connection (see Chapter 10) may be associated with a lower incidence of early postoperative arrhythmia. This has been attributed to less atrial distention, known to predispose to the initiation of atrial flutter in these patients (Figure 2). The long-term results in this

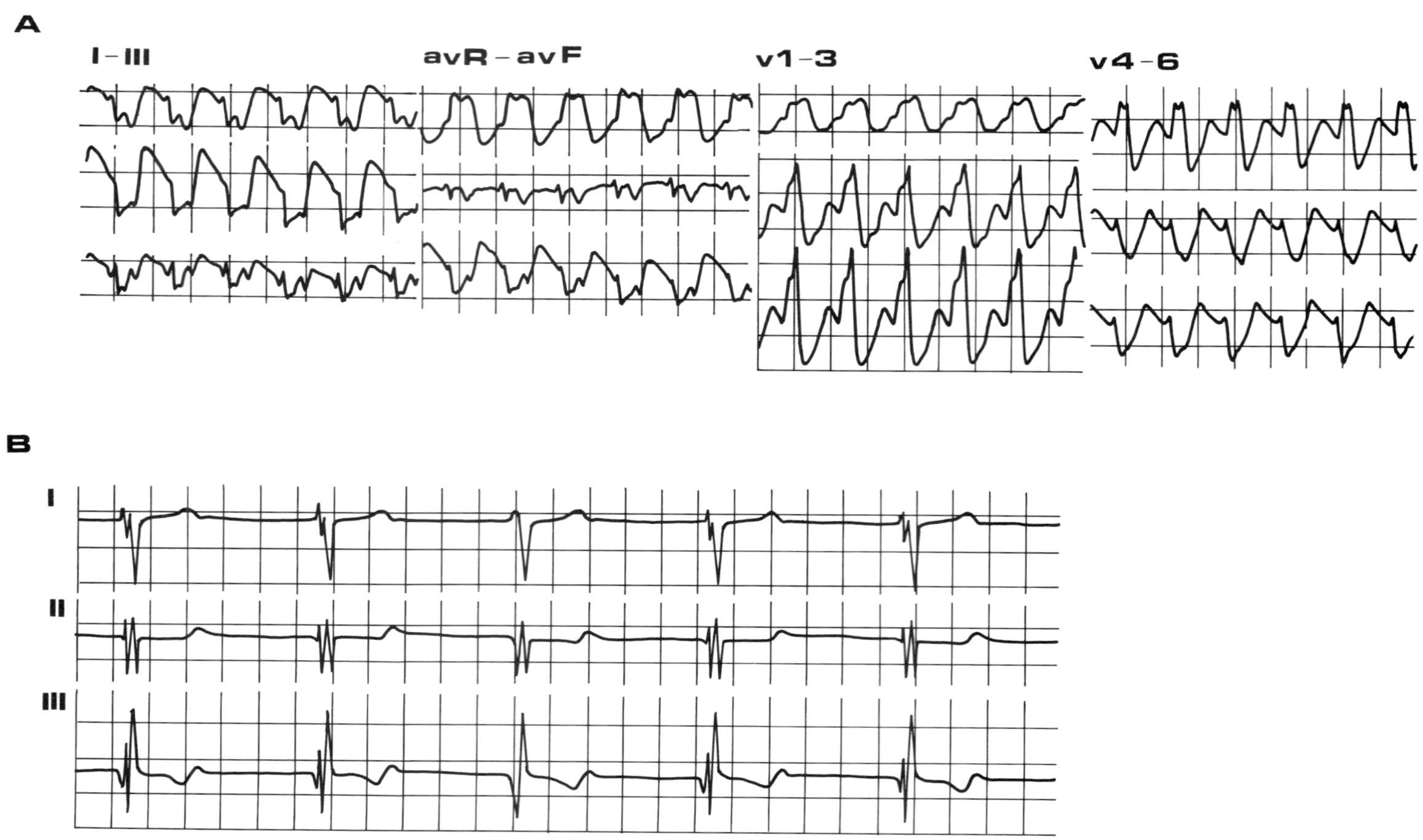

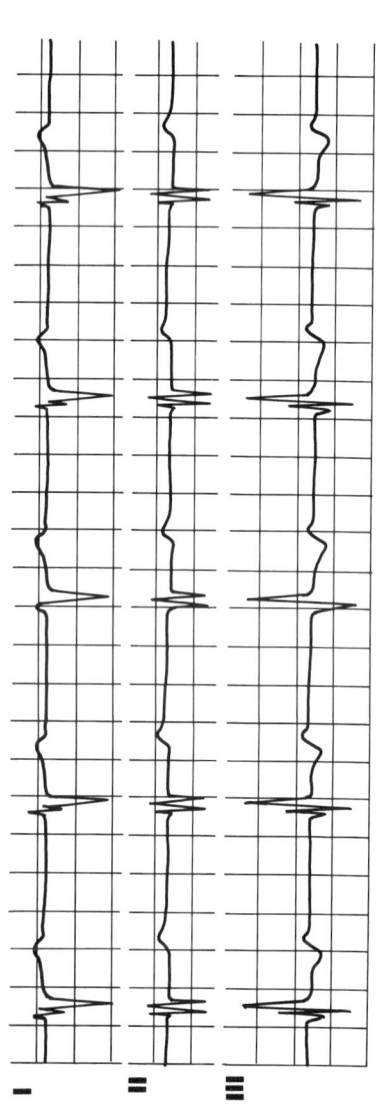

Figure 2. Atrial dysrhythmias after the Fontan procedure. (a) Shows atrial flutter with rate-related right bundle branch block. There was marked haemodynamic compromise. (b) Shows the same patient after spontaneous resolution of the tachycardia. There is a junctional escape rhythm which was haemodynamically much better tolerated.

group remain to be seen but the available data from those with atriopulmonary connection suggest an increase in prevalence of important arrhythmias with longer follow-up. Because of the adverse long-term effects of loss of sinus rhythm careful monitoring of all patients who have undergone a Fontan type operation is mandatory. Just as in patients after intra-atrial repair of transposition, the development of arrythmia makes haemodynamic evaluation mandatory, usually before treatment is started.

Bradyarrhythmias

It is a very rare patient indeed, that does not require permanent endocardial pacing for postoperative complete heart block due to direct trauma to the atrioventricular conduction tissue. This is not the only bradyarrythmia seen after surgery, however. Bradyarrhythmias may develop in any patient who has undergone congenital heart surgery. However, those in whom extensive atrial surgery has been performed are at greater risk. Thus, as with atrial tachyarrhythmias, patients after the Mustard operation are most at risk. Symptomatic bradycardia always requires treatment, but asymptomatic slow nodal rhythm is a more difficult clinical problem. An aggressive approach with pacemaker implantation has been advocated. However, in a number of large series in which this approach was adopted, it did not seem to reduce the incidence of late sudden death and many patients have died despite normally functioning pacemakers. This suggests that bradycardic sudden death is uncommon, and a more rigorous assessment for coexisting ventricular or atrial tachyarrhythmias may be more rewarding.

There are two other lesions associated with late development of heart block. Spontaneous complete heart block is common in congenitally corrected transposition (atrioventricular discordance, ventriculoarterial discordance). In one large series, 30% of 111 patients seen over a 20-year period at a single institution developed complete heart block. Much less common is 'spontaneous' heart block in patients after repair of primum atrial septal defect. A bifascicular block pattern, with a prolonged P–R interval is quite common, and does not require treatment but some of these patients develop complete heart block on follow-up. This is the main reason for continued regular outpatient review in this group.

Ventricular arrhythmias

The development of ventricular arrhythmias following repair of congenital heart defects can have a serious effect on long-term morbidity and mortality. However, the cause/effect relationship between development of ventricular arrhythmias and late sudden death is a source of much debate. Two conditions deserve special mention, namely aortic stenosis and tetralogy of Fallot.

Aortic Stenosis

Serious ventricular arrhythmias have been widely recognized in patients with severe aortic valve stenosis who have undergone surgery. In studies with long-term follow-up, residual elevated left ventricular end-diastolic pressure and cardiomegaly on chest X-ray (presumably related to aortic regurgitation) have been shown to be risk factors for the development of ventricular arrhythmias following surgical aortic valvotomy. Statistical analysis has estimated that an increase of left ventricular end-diastolic pressure by 5 mmHg can lead to doubling of the odds of developing serious arrhythmias. Patients who have undergone aortic valve replacement may be at even more risk. All in all, patients with severe aortic stenosis are more prone to develop ventricular arrhythmias than those with milder disease.

Tetralogy of Fallot

Almost all series with long-term follow-up after repair of tetralogy of Fallot have shown an incidence of late sudden death. Ambulatory electrocardiography may detect ventricular arrhythmias (greater than Lown grade 2) in up to 40–50% of patients (Figure 3). It has been suggested that the incidence increases with duration of follow-up. In most studies older age at the time of operation and residual high right ventricular systolic and end-diastolic pressures have been implicated. The ventriculotomy itself, placement of transannular patch and later development of pulmonary regurgitation all play a part, however. Some have advocated long-term prophylactic anti-arrhythmic therapy along with the use of aggressive electrophysiological studies to reduce the impact of ventricular arrhythmias and improve long-term survival, even in asymptomatic patients. However, there are no data available to support such an approach. There is little disagreement in the management of a symptomatic patient although the causal relationship between ventricular arrhythmia and late sudden death has not been established. It is worth noting, however, that asymptomatic ventricular arrhythmia is common following repair of tetralogy of Fallot, and late sudden death is rare.

Table 1.   Investigation of Patients with Suspected Arrhythmia

Detailed clinical examination
Standard 12-lead electrocardiogram
Ambulatory ECG monitoring
Formal exercise test
Cross-sectional echocardiography and Doppler examination
± Cardiac catheterization
± Formal electrophysiological study

I-III   aVR-aVF   V1-3   V4-6

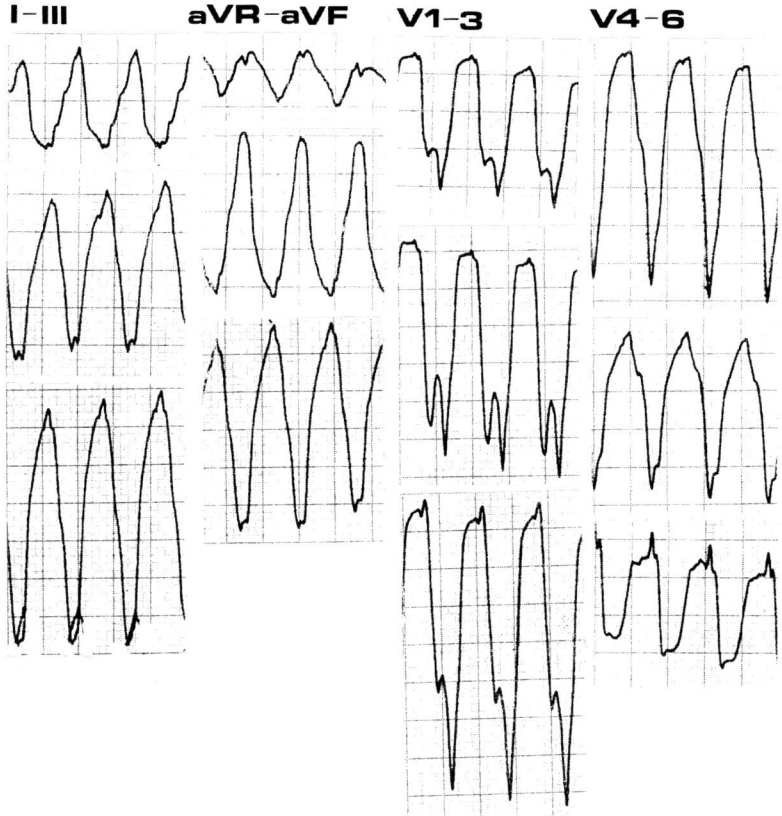

Figure 3. Sustained symptomatic ventricular tachycardia after tetralogy of Fallot. Treatment is clearly required. Non-sustained asymptomatic VT is much more common (see text for discussion).

Investigations (Table 1)

The most important prerequisite to the management of patients with late cardiac arrhythmia is accurate documentation of the arrhythmia on a 12-lead electro-cardiogram if possible. If intermittent, ambulatory electrocardiography may detect the arrhythmia although the lack of sensitivity and reproducibility of this investigation is well recognized. Clinical and haemodynamic assessment is indicated in all patients who have undergone cardiac surgery presenting with a new arrhythmia for the first time. Investigations include chest X-ray, detailed cross-sectional echocardiography with Doppler proceeding to cardiac catheter-ization if necessary. An example would be patients presenting with tachyarrhyth-mia following interatrial repair for transposition of the great arteries who may have severe venous pathway obstruction in the absence of major clinical findings. All patients require standard 12-lead electrocardiograms which should be compared to their initial postoperative ECGs if available and they may need ambulatory electrocardiography. Detailed electrophysiological study may be required but depends mainly on the type of rhythm disturbance and the availability of local facilities and expertise. They are notoriously difficult to interpret, as there is so little cross-sectional or longitudinal data for the various patient groups. With the increasing use of transcatheter electrophysiological interventions, e.g. radiofrequency ablation, it is likely that the number of patients undergoing therapeutic electrophysiological studies will increase.

Drug therapy

Assuming that a haemodynamic abnormality predisposing to the arrhythmia has been excluded, and that there are no other unrelated haemodynamic abnormalities, the treatment of these arrythmias follows conventional lines. It is an undocumented impression that proarrythmia may be more common in these patients, and as a rule, new agents should be introduced in hospital.

Key references

Deanfield J (1991) Late ventricular arrhythmias occurring after repair of tetralogy of Fallot: do they matter? *Int J Cardiol* **30**: 143–50.

Gewillig M, Cullen S, Mertens B, Lesaffre E, Deanfield J (1990) Risk factors for death after Mustard operation for simple transposition of the great arteries. *Circulation* **82** (suppl. III): 77 (abstract).

Vetter VL, Tanner CS, Horowitz LN (1987) Electrophysiologic consequences of the Mustard repair of d-transposition of the great arteries. *J Am Coll Cardiol* **6**: 1265–73.

Weber HS, Helenbrand WE, Kleinman CS, Perlmutter RA, Rosenfeld LE (1989) Predictors of rhythm disturbances and subsequent morbidity after the Fontan operation. *Am J Cardiol* **64**: 762–67.

27 Employment, Insurance and Driving

In collaboration with David S Celermajer

Introduction

Any young adults who survive with congenital heart disease may have important psychosocial difficulties, even if they are clinically well and stable. About 90% of patients with congenital heart disease who have reached adulthood are symptom-free and well, and these subjects expect a good quality of life. The other 10% often have haemodynamic and/or electrophysiological problems, which limit their day-to-day activities and their future prospects for a normal socioeconomic outcome. Employment prospects and insurability of these young adults are practical aspects of life about which many patients and their parents have concern. The American Heart Association has now published recommendations on life insurance and health insurance, but few guidelines exist elsewhere. In the United Kingdom, a recent survey has shown that most young adults with congenital heart disease are only insurable at high rates or, in the case of many lesions, not insurable at all.

Employability of young adults with congenital heart disease may be based on their current clinical state, the likely sickness and absence record, possible premature termination of career and aspects of pension planning. In the United States, the National Rehabilitation Act of 1973 has improved the employment prospects for any patient with a handicap, as emphasis is placed on the present capacity of a person to perform a particular task rather than on projections of future deterioration; no such law exists in Britain. Employment policy is therefore somewhat variable, and this results in some inconsistencies in the attitudes and practices of prospective employers.

Insurance

Health insurance

Few data are available on the proportion of young adults with congenital heart disease who have health insurance, and the data are difficult to interpret because of the wide variation of government-subsidized and private health insurance schemes that exist in different countries. In the recent NHS-2 survey of American children with aortic stenosis, pulmonary stenosis and ventricular septal defect who survived into adult life, approximately 15% of patients reported having no health insurance, compared to 12% of controls. Therefore the proportion of uninsured adults with congenital heart disease was slightly but not significantly higher than the national figures. It is possible that subjects with more complex congenital heart defects may have lower rates of health insurance coverage, particularly those who are unemployed and therefore would not be eligible for group coverage.

In the United States medical expenses incurred during childhood are often covered by a parent's private insurance or by a public programme such as Crippled Children's Services or Medicaid. Such insurance will lapse at the age of 19 years, unless the insured is a full-time student or remains eligible for Medicaid coverage because of low income. Crippled Children's Services will not support patients' health costs when they are over 21 years. Costs incurred for young adults include those associated with clinic visits, hospitalizations, medication, doctors' fees and hospital charges. These costs may be significant, and may cause serious financial embarrassment to those who cannot obtain private health insurance, particularly those who require open heart surgery. Among several recommendations that have been made by the American Heart Association 5th Conference on Insurability are the concepts that the insurance industry should re-establish community rating, with the public accepting the need to insure not only themselves but others with established serious illness.

In the United Kingdom and other countries with a government-sponsored national health service, all adults with congenital heart disease are covered. However, private health insurance, to enable access to a doctor of choice in a private clinic, is severely restricted for patients with congenital heart disease. Private insurance is usually available until the age of 18 or 21 years under a family policy. However, after this, a policy would be underwritten to exclude any future benefit for medical or surgical treatment of the heart condition.

Life insurance

Overall, approximately 35% of the NHS-2 participants had no life insurance, compared to a national average of approximately 32%. These young adults with relatively mild congenital heart defects represent the best end of the spectrum and again, it is reasonable to assume that those with more complex congenital heart defects will have lower rates of life insurance. Life insurability of adults with congenital heart disease in the United States has been studied in detail by Truesdell et al, and many lesions are uninsurable or insurable at high premiums only. The results of a similar survey in the United Kingdom have also recently become available (Table 1). Many insurance companies and doctors in Britain refer to data on medical selection of life risks compiled by Breckenridge, who suggests that most subjects with complex congenital heart disease are uninsurable, and that many with simple lesions can only be insured at high rating. Some of the current British recommendations seem unduly harsh on the basis of available data concerning the natural history; for example, young adults with mild pulmonary stenosis and those who have had successful repair of small atrial or ventricular septal defects appear to have an excellent long-term prognosis. In contrast, some other ratings may be generous, such as normal rate insurance for postoperative coarctation of the aorta, given the recognized hazard for early mortality in large series (Chapter 13). Follow-up studies for patients with more complex heart disease are of much shorter duration, as effective surgical treatment may have only recently become available. Inconsistencies between life insurance companies were also noted, and young adults declined by one company should make enquiries at several others at which they may be insurable, albeit at high rates. Inability to get life insurance may be a serious disadvantage to a young adult who is married and may have dependent children. In Britain, most mortgage companies require applicants to hold life insurance as suitable collateral for a long-term loan, and therefore an inability to obtain life insurance may also preclude the purchase of a new home.

One factor that often influences insurance prospects is the severity of the disorder, as assessed by the subject's physician. Patients with mild valve disease may well be eligible for life insurance whereas those with moderate or severe disease might be declined. In view of this, accurate grading of such lesions is of great importance. Clearly, as more data on the natural history of congenital heart lesions becomes available, rational life insurance decisions will become possible. As insurance companies are fiscally conservative, however, many young adults with congenital heart disease can expect difficulties getting standard life insurance coverage, until much longer-term survival data becomes available.

Employment

In the NHS-2 study of long-term follow-up of adults with simple congenital heart diseases, approximately 75% were currently employed, 10% were students, 5% were housewives and 10% were unemployed. Within each defect group, those managed surgically rather than medically were more likely to be students or to be unemployed. These figures were not significantly different from the

Table 1. Life insurability of congenital heart defects

Defect	Normal	High rates	Decline
Aortic regurgitation			
mild		*	
moderate		*	
severe			*
Aortic stenosis			
mild		*	
moderate			*
severe			*
Mitral regurgitation			
mild		*	
moderate		*	
severe			*
Mitral stenosis			
mild		*	
moderate		*	
severe			*
Mitral valve prolapse (no regurgitation)	*		
Mitral valve replacement		*(1)	
Aortic valve replacement		*(1)	
Double valve replacement			*
Pulmonary stenosis			
mild		*	
moderate		*	
severe			*
Ebsteins's			
mild			*
moderate			*
severe			*
postoperative			*
Atrial septal defect			
pulmonary to systemic shunt <2		*	
pulmonary to systemic shunt ≥2		*	
pulmonary to systemic shunt postoperative		*(2)	
Ventricular septal defect			
pulmonary to systemic shunt <2		*	
pulmonary to systemic shunt >2		*	
pulmonary to systemic shunt postoperative			
normal		*(2)	
pulmonary to systemic shunt postoperative			
↑ pulmonary vascular resistance			*
Patent arterial duct			
preoperative			*
postoperative	*		
Coarctation of aorta			
mild			*
moderate			*
severe			*(3)
postoperative normal	*		
postoperative ↑ blood pressure		*	

Defect	Normal	High rates	Decline
Tetralogy of Fallot			
preoperative		*	
postoperative		*(4)	
Transposition of the great arteries			
post-Mustard/Senning			*
post-arterial switch			*(5)
Total anomalous pulmonary venous return			
postoperative		*	
Truncus			
postoperative			*
Fontan procedure			*
Congenital complete heart block	*		

Notes:
1. Policy limited to 25 years' postoperative by one company.
2. Reducing to normal rates after 4 years by two companies.
3. High-rate policy limited to 50 years of age by one company.
4. High-rate policy for short duration only by two companies.
5. High-rate policy for limited duration by one company.
↑ Indicates raised value.

national average. However, among the patients whose clinical status was judged to be poor, less than half were employed.

In the recent British survey of employer policies, respondents from 14 British companies were generally optimistic about job prospects for young adults with simple or totally corrected heart defects, but less favourably disposed to those with complex or only partially corrected problems. Furthermore, it is very difficult for a young adult with any congenital heart disease to gain employment in the armed services. Otherwise, employability was usually based on a functional assessment at the time of application, occasionally a report from the applicant's physician, and/or consideration of the future prospects for absenteeism and premature death or ill-health in midlife. Overall, one can be optimistic regarding employers' attitudes to patients, and employability is rarely a major issue in these patients.

Driving and flying

There are several occupations in which the safety of work colleagues or members of the general public may be endangered if patients at risk of sudden disability or death are employed. Therefore separate recommendations for driving and flying are available for young adults with congenital heart disease.

Rational recommendations about fitness to drive heavy goods or public service vehicles or to fly aircraft ideally requires a comparison of the risk of major morbid events, such as serious arrhythmia or stroke and sudden death, with age- and sex-matched controls. This remains difficult with regard to congenital heart disease, mainly because the maximum postoperative follow-up period is still only 35–40 years. For many prospective employees, this time period does not yet cover the duration of their potential career. Furthermore, over this period there have been substantial improvements in medical and surgical practice, including improved myocardial protection and bypass techniques, better diagnosis, and the development of improved operative procedures. Therefore, the survival data that are available from this early era are perhaps not applicable to children who are treated today.

The current British recommendations for driving a heavy goods or public service vehicle excludes young adults with certain types of cardiac defect. Those ineligible include patients with paroxysmal arrhythmia, the presence of a cardiac pacing device, the presence of a bioprosthetic valve or conduit and patients on medication to treat heart failure. For flying, conditions with an estimated event rate $<1\%$ per annum for multicrew flights or $<0.1\%$ per annum for solo flights have been approved for prospective pilots. Therefore lesions potentially compatible with certification to fly include repaired atrial septal defect or arterial duct, repaired pulmonary stenosis and repaired coarctation of the aorta, as long as surgery took place under the age of 14 years and the current blood pressure is normal. Multicrew licences might be available for patients with mild aortic stenosis or repaired ventricular septal defect.

Conclusion

As the paediatric cardiac successes of the modern era reach adulthood, they face problems of both a medical and social nature. One of the most important measures of a successful outcome is the ability to find gainful employment and health and life insurance. Although many young adults with simple and corrected defects may obtain insurance and employment, prospects are less good for those with complex defects or residual postoperative problems. As congenital heart surgery becomes more adventurous and postoperative care results in even better outcomes, more patients with complex anatomy will be reaching adult life, and posing challenges for their physicians in terms of optimizing both their medical and socioeconomic outcome. As data on natural and postoperative survival become available, guidelines for employers and insurers should be devised. The absence of such guidelines will occasionally disadvantage patients inappropriately. One of the major roles for specialized centres for the care of young adults with congenital heart disease is to have a role in defining functional capacity and long-term survival prospects of this group, as well as the important task of aiding individual patients in their search for both employment and insurance.

Key references

AHA committee report (1980) Guidelines for insurability of patients with congenital heart disease. *Circulation* **62**: 1419A–24A.

Allen HD, Gersony WM, Taubert KA (1992) Insurability of the adolescent and young adult with heart disease. *Circulation* **86**: 703–10.

Celermajer DS, Deanfield JE (1993) Employment and insurance for young adults with congenital heart disease. *Br Heart J* **69**: 539–43.

Moller JH, Anderson RC (1992) Natural history of congenital heart disease. 1000 consecutive children with cardiac malformations with 26–37-year follow-up. *Am J Cardiol* **70**: 661–67.

Recommendations of the Secretary of State's Honorary Medical Advisory Panel concerning cardiac conditions and drivers of heavy good vehicles and public service vehicles (1989) *Government General Health Trends*, leaflet CLEIII.

Report from the Joint Study on the Natural History of Congenital Heart Defects. *Circulation* **87** (suppl. I): 1–126.

Truesdell SC, Skorton DJ, Laver RM (1986) Life insurance for children with cardiovascular disease. *Paediatrics* **77**: 687–91.

Index

Tables in **bold**
Figures in *italic*